'In this major achievement Dr. Robbins demonstrates the sweep of his scholarship in a stunning analysis of the human difference from other species with regard to mental structure, civilisation and destructiveness. He integrates psychoanalysis with evolution theory, primatology and sociology and examines manifestations of human destructiveness that have no parallel in other species such as murder, war, persecution and devastation of the environment related to the explosive increase in human population.'

Henry Lothane, *clinical professor of Psychiatry, Icahn School of Medicine*

'Robbins penetrates the mystery of the leap from body to mind and explores the origins of civilisation and malignant human destructiveness. He explains Freud's limited understanding of biology and introduces the role of neoteny and dependency on caregivers in the acquisition of a second mental process unique to humans. His experience in treating the psychoses helps Robbins to revise the theory of evolution and integrate it with psychoanalytic theory, offering a deeper understanding of human nature. Original and fascinating!'

Riccardo Lombardi, MD, *author of* Body-Mind Dissociation in Psychoanalysis *and* Formless Infinity

THE HUMAN DIFFERENCE

From a multidisciplinary perspective grounded in psychoanalysis, this book explores the manifestations of mind that distinguish humans from other species: culture, civilization, and destructiveness.

Psychoanalysis was created by Freud in an effort to understand neurosis and psychosis, the names he gave to individual human destructiveness. His understanding was limited and incorrect because the science of evolution and the disciplines of sociology and cultural anthropology were in their infancy when he formulated his ideas. He did not comprehend that destructiveness is qualitatively different in humans than in other species, and he ignored the problem of how biological instincts become mental processes. These limitations left psychoanalysis with one of its most perplexing unsolved problems, the mysterious leap from mind to body. This book explains how neoteny, the prolonged period of postnatal immaturity that distinguishes humans from other animals, requires and enables complex learning from caregivers. It is the knowledge acquired from this learning and its intergenerational transmission that links the biological theory of evolution with the psychosocial theory of psychoanalysis and explains how the human species is unique.

This book will be of interest to those who want to learn about how integrating the findings of evolutionary science, primatology, sociology, and cultural anthropology with the theory of psychoanalysis expands our understanding of what makes humans unique and its implications for the future of our species, and how it empowers us to influence the destiny of humankind.

Michael Robbins is a psychoanalyst, member of the American and International Psychoanalytic Societies, former professor of Clinical Psychiatry at Harvard Medical School, and author of 5 previous books and more than 40 articles in refereed journals.

THE HUMAN DIFFERENCE

Evolution, Civilization – and Destruction

Michael Robbins

Routledge
Taylor & Francis Group
LONDON AND NEW YORK

Designed cover image: A Mokhtari © Getty Images

First published 2024
by Routledge
4 Park Square, Milton Park, Abingdon, Oxon OX14 4RN

and by Routledge
605 Third Avenue, New York, NY 10158

Routledge is an imprint of the Taylor & Francis Group, an informa business

British Library Cataloguing-in-Publication Data
A catalogue record for this book is available from the British Library

Library of Congress Cataloging-in-Publication Data
Names: Robbins, Michael, M.D, author.
Title: The human difference : evolution, civilization, and destruction / Michael Robbins.
Description: Abingdon, Oxon ; New York, Ny : Routledge, 2024. | Includes bibliographical references and index. |
Identifiers: LCCN 2023018398 (print) | LCCN 2023018399 (ebook) | ISBN 9781032569444 (hardback) | ISBN 9781032580555 (paperback) | ISBN 9781003442318 (ebook)
Subjects: LCSH: Psychoanalysis and evolution. | Self-destructive behavior. | Freud, Sigmund, 1856-1939.
Classification: LCC BF175.4.E86 R63 2024 (print) | LCC BF175.4.E86 (ebook) | DDC 150.19/5—dc23/eng/20230627
LC record available at https://lccn.loc.gov/2023018398
LC ebook record available at https://lccn.loc.gov/2023018399

ISBN: 9781032569444 (hbk)
ISBN: 9781032580555 (pbk)
ISBN: 9781003442318 (ebk)

DOI: 10.4324/9781003442318

Typeset in Optima
by codeMantra

To three deceased men who profoundly influenced my professional development: James Winn, a high school teacher who took an interest in a clueless young man; Robert Grose, psychology professor at Amherst College; and Elvin Semrad, who was so effective reducing psychoanalysis to living and loving that I and many of my fellow graduate students in clinical psychology at Harvard defected to go to medical school and become psychoanalysts, and as a consequence Harvard fired him.

To sleep: perchance to dream: aye, there's the rub; For in that sleep of death what dreams may come when we have shuffled off this mortal coil must give us pause…

Hamlet, Act 3, Scene 1

CONTENTS

PREFACE

This is the second of two volumes devoted to the mental complexity that distinguishes homo sapiens from other species. The first book, *What Makes Humans Unique* (in press), is devoted to the foundation of the human mind – two intelligent mental structures: one present at birth that we share with other species and a second mental structure unique to humans, reflective representational thought, that has emerged in the course of human evolution and that develops in each of us during the course of maturation. This book focuses on the individual and social manifestations of this structural complexity and their implications for the human species. The two books integrate the findings of evolution, primatology, sociology, and cultural anthropology with the theory of psychoanalysis and expand the scope, power, and usefulness of each.

This book describes the manifestations of the human mind that set it apart from that of other species as a consequence of the acquisition of the second mental structure. We are justly proud of the creations known as culture and civilization. The book focuses on a less understood and appreciated dark side. Manifestations of the extent, depth, and virulence of human destructiveness are in our faces every day, but most of us would prefer to ignore their centrality in human life, and their origins and implications are not well understood. Freud created the discipline of psychoanalysis to study and treat individual destructiveness. He thought of it as mental illness, neurosis, and psychosis. Because the science of evolution was in its infancy when he formulated his theory, his understanding of evolution was limited, and he based his understanding of human destructiveness on several incorrect assumptions. He believed all creatures have a similar instinct to destroy themselves and he did not comprehend that human destructiveness is qualitatively different from that of other species. He glossed over the problem of how biological forces become mental processes, leaving psychoanalysis with one of its most perplexing unsolved problems – the mysterious leap from mind to body. This volume situates the psychoanalytic understanding of destructiveness in a multidisciplinary context that includes its social and species manifestations and insights gained from the century of additional understanding of evolution since his death.

A hitherto overlooked aspect of the biological theory of evolution known as neoteny helps to understand the human difference from other species and the unique nature and manifestations of human destructiveness in particular. It refers to the prolonged period of postnatal immaturity and dependency on caregivers that distinguishes humans from other animals. This prolonged postnatal immaturity requires and enables complex learning from caregivers and the development of a second mental process. It is the knowledge acquired from this learning and its intergenerational transmission that links the biological theory of evolution and the psychosocial theory of psychoanalysis. It makes it necessary to include the findings of psychoanalysis in the theory of evolution, and enables us to understand the uniqueness of human destructiveness from a psychoanalytic perspective.

1

INTRODUCTION

The mutually enriching contributions of the psychoanalytic theory of mind and the biological theory of evolution to understanding the uniqueness of human civilization and human destructiveness

The human mind is unique insofar as it has enabled the creation of an historical record of the evolution of its extraordinary creation, civilization, and culture. The darker side of this history that distinguishes us from other species is that humans have been extraordinarily destructive to ourselves and to one another, and we have formed social organizations that are destructive and ones that conflict with others that we form. This book explores these human creations, civilization, and destruction, with special emphasis on destructiveness, from the perspectives of two major disciplines – evolutionary biology that tells us how we got to be who we are as a species and the psychoanalytic theory of mind that explores how the human mind, which makes us different from other species, functions.

Evolutionary biology and psychoanalytic theory of mind have historically been separate disciplines, isolated from one another. This book and the companion volume *What Makes Humans Unique: Evolution and the Structures of Mind* (in press) demonstrate a fundamental relationship between them and show how each discipline has critical information to contribute to the other and to our understanding of how and why humans are different from other species. The mutual enrichment that can result from this realization can lead to the growth and expansion of each field. While describing the implications of a psychoanalytic understanding of mind for the theory of evolution, this book concentrates on the hitherto neglected significance of biological aspects of evolution for psychoanalysis as a theory and for our understanding of human beings, human society, and the fate of the human species.

Why and how is the theory of evolution critical to broadening the scope and application of psychoanalysis to individuals, society, and our species? What is the particular importance of evolutionary biology to understanding

DOI: 10.4324/9781003442318-1

a problem psychoanalysis has mostly avoided trying to grapple with – the unusual extent, depth, and virulence of human destructiveness?

Of less immediate importance to psychoanalysis, but of great importance to biological science, is another question. Why and how is understanding the origin and nature of the human mind, and especially its difference from that of other species including our nearest primate kin, critically important to broadening the theory of evolution to take into account psychosocial causation, without abandoning its biological foundation?

Freud's limiting definition of the scope, parameters, and basic assumptions of the psychoanalytic exploration of mind in relation to biology and to destructiveness continues to constrain the scope and utility of psychoanalysis. His background was in the nineteenth century equivalent of neuroscience, and he was acutely aware of the neurobiological roots of mind when he formulated his theories. He wrote:

> The deficiencies in our experience would probably vanish if we were already in a position to replace the psychological terms by physiological or chemical ones...we may expect it [biology] to give us the most surprising information and we cannot guess what answers it will return in a few dozen years to the questions we have put to it.
>
> *(1920, p. 60)*

He understood that mental processes were driven by biological instincts, but his way of conceptualizing the process was limited in ways that have had profound consequences for psychoanalysis. He conceived of an underlying biological life force (Eros) and another destructive counterforce toward death or entropy (Thanatos). He seems to have been unaware of the problem of how a biological process becomes something uniquely human – a mental idea. Instead, he made what Felix Deutsch (1963) and many others felicitously called "the mysterious leap," from the body, biology, to the mind, psychology. He postulated a psychic representation of Eros, the instinct to preserve and enhance life, in the form of what he called a libidinal drive, conceived of as wish. He further postulated a struggle between both drives, toward wish-fulfillment and destructive aggression, and the clash of these drives with civilizing authority.

Klein made a similar unsubstantiated assumption about the innate biological origins of destructiveness and formulated a theory in which the fundamental force behind human development is a biological death instinct, experienced psychologically from the moment of birth as rage, and early development involves infantile efforts to combat and control it.

Freud made another incorrect assumption about biology and human nature, that all animal species are biologically driven by similar life and death/destruction counterforces. In his time, neither zoology (especially primatology) nor sociobiology was developed disciplines, and he was unaware that the destructiveness in humans is not qualitatively similar to that in other species. It is much more virulent, deep, and extensive. This lack of awareness is particularly puzzling considering that the discipline of psychoanalysis that he conceived of is an attempt to comprehend the origins and nature of human destructiveness, neurotic, psychotic, and characterological, pathologies that are not encountered in other species, except at times when animals are removed from their natural habitat and held captive in human environments such as zoos. Neurosis and psychosis are destructive to individual human beings and often lead to inflicting subtle or overt harm on other individuals or on society. And while he was well aware of the human difference from other species with regard to culture and civilization, he did not wonder whether and how that difference might also relate to biology.

It is not accurate to say that Freud turned his back on the human difference, particularly destructiveness. In his famous WWII dialogue with Einstein, *Why War*, he was quite pessimistic about human destructiveness. However, he and others followed in the footsteps of Carl Linnaeus, the evolutionary taxonomist who optimistically named our species homo sapiens in recognition of our "higher order" difference from other species. It has been easier to look at the achievements of human creativity in isolation from biology than to consider the dark side of the human difference and its unique biological connection. Our species might just as well have merited the designation homo destrudo, borrowing the term coined by Eduardo Weiss (1942), who elaborated Freud's concept of a death instinct.

True to its inherent identity as a discipline that studies destructive aspects of mind, psychoanalysis has not been content with this avoidance. The discipline of neuro-psychoanalysis, which attempts to bridge the gap between body and mind, has grown in popularity in recent decades. And countless clinicians and analysts, some of whose work is cited throughout the book, have studied individual and social destructiveness beyond Freud's model of socialization conflicts involving libidinal wish-fulfillment. However, like Freud's theory of neurotic conflict and development of symptoms, inhibitions, diffuse anxieties, and character deformations, the psychoanalysis of destructiveness has not been convincingly linked to biology and the question of what makes humans different from other species.

Evolutionary biology has also avoided confronting the knotty problem of human difference from other species. It has not accounted for the uniquely human development of reflective representational thinking and the civilization, culture, as well as the unusual destructiveness that makes humans different. This avoidance began quite unintentionally in Darwin's time because the data he and others chose to study, for reasons of convenience portability, consisted of small plants and insects, and from this extrapolations were made to large systems; whole animals like humans. More recently, since the work of Gregor Mendel, this kind of avoidance has been perpetuated by the opening of the exciting new visa of micro and molecular biology and the study of genetics, genes, and DNA.

The kinds of destructiveness found among humans have little or no parallel in other species. Human destructiveness is an increasingly pressing problem, one to which psychoanalysis has a standing invitation to substantially contribute. In the preface to his important 1973 effort to shed some new light on this problem, Erich Fromm writes that the study of destructiveness is "one of the fundamental theoretical problems in psychoanalysis…[and]…the wave of destructiveness engulfing the world makes it also one of the most practically relevant ones" (brackets mine). If this was true half a century ago, during the Vietnam War, it is exponentially the case now.

Even allowing for the media penchant for conflating violence and horror with "news" that will sell the most papers and attract the most TV viewers, it is difficult to escape the conclusion that humans have a remarkable penchant for destruction that sets us apart from other living things every bit as much as our more "civilized" accomplishments. We wring our figurative hands about global warming due to greenhouse gas emissions, leading to melting glaciers, rising sea levels, uncontrolled wildfires, extremes of weather that endanger human life, and tropical forests turning into barren deserts. We observe with horror the extinction of other species by human hands. We worry about war and the threat of war, the consequences of nuclear weapon proliferation. We lament the latest acts of terrorism and violence and debate gun control. We watch in horror a terrorist group invade and try to destroy the peaceful congress of a society attempting to democratically elect a new leader. The catalog of destructiveness, elaborated in the next chapter, is horrifying.

Self-destructive behavior is common in other animal species, but sociobiologists have discovered that its individual nature appears to have a selective, constructive evolutionary purpose in relation to survival, propagation, and equilibration of the group, in contrast to the random, senseless destruction to individuals, social organization, and species survival found in homo sapiens.

Furthermore, the phenomenology that comprises human destructiveness is not so obvious as it seemed to Freud and to many others who have studied the problem. In determining what constitutes human destructiveness, it is necessary to compare and contrast homo sapiens with other species and to highlight qualitative distinctions. In so doing, it becomes apparent that some of the developments we think of as creative, civilized, and progressive may have a darker side if viewed from another context. Many of these are consequences of another uniquely human development, the evolution of social organization based on individual self-actualization. They include such things as social conflict based on clashes of belief systems and their leaders, technology, and "advances" that have served to preserve and enhance individual life and in so doing fueled an unchecked population explosion that threatens the continuing vitality of our planet and its non-human inhabitants. Consider an example of the human leap from simple primate abilities to sophisticated social-cultural accomplishments. Chimps use natural environmentally available objects as spears and clubs to kill prey they need for food, but despite evidence of hand and mouth conflict between males for territorial control, there is no evidence from their instrumental repertory or their social behavior of anything resembling the human propensity to perceive members of other species as dangerous and create conflict and war with them, much less to be able to develop technology to do it. In WWII, the Nazis concluded people living on an island far removed were an enemy, invented the V-2 rocket, and blitzed London. And the United States invented nuclear weapons and delivered the bomb thousands of miles by airplane to devastate cities on a distant island. Chimp collectives seem only to try to perpetuate themselves, not to expand in size, take over other colonies, or create an advanced civilization.

If human destructiveness is qualitatively different from that of other species, then it is logical to assume that there must be something equally unique about its evolution and ask how such a phenomenon might have come about.

Darwin assumed evolution is a biologically driven process common to all species. He focused for the most part on small collectable botanical specimens where, at least as it was then understood, there was no problem of mind and thought to consider. Other evolutionary scientists followed in his footsteps and included insects and birds. Recent developments tend to focus on microbiology, the study of genes, DNA, and their evolution, independent of the organisms that bear them. Despite recent interest from cultural anthropologists, the complexities of human mind, socio-cultural development, and even destructiveness have not evoked the attention from students of evolution that they deserve. Human evolution is still believed to involve the process of natural selection of genes responsible for the phenotypes most likely to survive. But it is not easy to make the case that the nature, extent, and virulence of human destructiveness makes the human species uniquely fit to survive.

In the late 1800s, attempts to account for the human difference turned to the possible evolutionary value of the attributes that make our species unique: socialized learning, civilization, and culture. Biologically oriented theorists traced its origins to mutations that are the underpinnings of speech, language, communication, and socialized learning. A theory known as gene-culture coevolution or dual inheritance was developed to account for transmission of social-cultural learning and accumulation of knowledge. Richerson and Boyd (2006) proposed what they called the theory of gene-culture coevolution, or dual inheritance theory, that the biological and the social-cultural comprise a complex system with emergent properties. They give such examples as the evolution of the human brain and vocal apparatus, changes that, in turn, enable social communication and learning and therefore create phenotypes that favor survival and hence are selectively transmitted and perpetuated. However much they take important note of social and cultural factors, theirs is still a basically biological theory of evolution. And in ignoring the extent and virulence of human destructiveness, they avoid confronting the question of whether this unique aspect of human beings favors or threatens survival of the species. A similar hypothesis is advanced by Henrich (2015). He proposes that cultural evolution makes humans unique and that its defining characteristic is social learning; the capacity to learn from one another. However, he operates within a Darwinian framework insofar as he believes this cultural learning is transmitted through genetic perpetuation of this adaptive phenotype, and in doing so, he does not ask whether such a phenotype actually favors survival.

However, it is not clear that somatic changes that enhanced communication and socialization brought about by acquisition of speech of themselves have enhanced the survival prospects of the human species. After all, humans talk about all sorts of things and socialize in ways that sometimes seem constructive and other times not. And in the broader sense, it is difficult to imagine how the extent, depth, and virulence of human destructiveness is even compatible with species survival, much less with enhancing it.

The gulf that comprises the human difference remains one that theory has yet to successfully bridge. The key to closing the gap may reside in an insufficiently appreciated biological difference known as neoteny, the lengthy period of maturation required after birth that distinguishes humans from even our closest primate kin. Members of other species, even our closest primate ancestors, are mature and functionally independent either at birth, or relatively soon thereafter. They are born with a genetically preprogrammed mental process common to all sentient species and rapidly attain species maturity and a functional independence that is largely reflexive and biologically driven. Their minds do not develop further than what is reflexively necessary to ensure survival in the immediate environments they inhabit. While they never transcend the primordial biologically programmed mental process with which they are born, some species seem more sophisticated in its use than others. Humans, in contrast, require approximately two decades of dependence on caregivers before reaching full maturity and independence. But neoteny does not in itself account for the human difference. During the prolonged period of immaturity, human young are required to depend on and learn from caregivers, who themselves have learned from other caregivers and are products of their particular historical era, society, and culture. As part of that learning process, we develop a second mental process, reflective representational thought, which leads to acquisition of the knowledge and creativity we call civilization, but also to destructive tendencies unknown to other species. We imagine and often create worlds beyond our immediate concrete surroundings. The knowledge we acquire and accumulate, in turn, is transmitted by teaching and learning to subsequent generations, and it grows in scope and complexity independent of our biology and functions to some extent independently of our immediate surroundings. This, in essence, comprises the human difference, an autonomous psychosocial evolutionary force, but one that depends on the uniqueness of human biology. Reflective thought does not replace primordial mentation but is more adaptive in many situations in mature adult life and is responsible for civilization and its discontents. Although the reflective thought that distinguishes humans is responsible for the achievements of civilization of which we take pride, it does not make us the superior altruistic socially cooperative progressively improving species that has transcended many of the problems of life and death that eventually doom other species, that many philosophers from the past and contemporary theorists and journalists wish to believe.

The lengthy period of human immaturity and dependency on caregivers that is responsible for the unique development of reflective thought brings with it the risk of pathological development and learning that leads to destructiveness. Children who have been psychologically damaged by parents and others during the attachment-separation phase of early development become adults who, in turn, damage their children, and this unfortunate product of learned intergenerational transmission is responsible for individual self-destructiveness that is unparalleled in other species.

During the course of human evolution, the sociocentric tribal structures typical of other primates and of earliest human social organization, in which individual members function as cogs or parts that seem to serve the function of maintaining social equilibrium and stability, have gradually been replaced by self-centric social structures based on care and enhancement of individual persons. Much of human destructiveness is the result of things we ordinarily think of as creative, constructive, and progressive because they appear to enhance individual lives, though if we look closely, such "selfishness" is not always constructive for human social organization or for the planet as a whole. In the process social groupings based on self-interest also promote human social conflict, are destructive to other species and the environment, and lead to an uncontrolled growth of human population that may have potentially lethal consequences for the species. One example is the domestication of animals, an evolutionary development dating back thousands of years, which has had vast destructive consequences related to things like population expansion, conflict among groups, and destruction of species integrity and the environment.

Looked at from the perspective of our species as a whole, some of our relatively recent and most valued human accomplishments designed to preserve and enhance individual lives, attributable to science, medicine, and public health, are responsible for an explosion of population unprecedented in human history and unparalleled in other species. The average lifespan has doubled or tripled since the Middle Ages. The human population is estimated to have been approximately one billion around 1700. By 1900, after several hundred years of industrial revolution and in the early stages of the remarkable developments in science and medicine, it had reached one billion six hundred million. In 1927 it reached two billion, and in 1950, 2.5 billion. Now, less than 75 years later, it has skyrocketed to what the UN has estimated as eight billion. The consequences of this astonishing and uncontrolled development have not been sufficiently noted and appreciated. Overpopulation generates social conflict and leads to destruction and depletion of scarce resources as well as destruction of other species, and therein threatens the planet on which we depend as well as our own continuity as a species.

The medical response to the current COVID-19 pandemic is a recent example of human success preserving otherwise endangered human life. Our focus on reducing individual mortality, developing new ways to treat infected individuals, public health measures to contain the spread of the illness, and developing vaccines to immunize otherwise susceptible persons has led to a change in outcome from previous pandemics. In "darker" ages, such a pandemic might have reduced earth's population to a more sustainable size, as happened periodically, for instance, with plagues that recurred throughout history until very recently. Now, pandemics are little more than detours in the road of inexorable population growth.

The Greek myth of Prometheus tells of punishments inflicted on humans for acts of hubris. The Book of Genesis in the Judeo-Christian Bible attributes the primal sin and fall from grace to the acquisition of knowledge. Perhaps that apple contained the internet or the knowledge to construct a nuclear reactor or artificial intelligence. According to Abrahamic religious scripture, God created all life but may have made a mistake endowing humans with the unique capacity to learn and acquire knowledge. Such stories remarkably parallel the challenge homo sapiens poses to what appears to have been the natural order of things among species prior to our advent. Perhaps "man" has had the arrogance to aspire to be immortal like the Gods. The prospect of everlasting life, hitherto imaginable only in mythology, has fueled much scientific research as well as literature such as George Bernard Shaw's *Back to Methuselah* series, asking, among other things, what would humans become if we could live indefinitely?

The human difference, reflective representational thought, has led to a complex combination of soaring creative achievements and deadly destructiveness, as well as manifestations that seem constructive if viewed from one perspective but destructive from another. The constructive achievements are not only referred to throughout the book, but are implicit in the book itself; reading, writing, communicating at a distance, discussing subjects beyond the moment that have to do with an historical past, an imagined future, and problems. Freud created the discipline of psychoanalysis to explore aspects of human destructiveness that are not encountered in other species, and the discussion to come is an attempt to enlarge the psychoanalytic discourse to embrace the unique extent, depth, and virulence of human destructiveness, that comprises a remarkable manifestation of the human difference that has been insufficiently studied. Such an investigation might empower psychoanalysis to assume a critically important role in comprehending and hopefully fundamentally mitigating some of the problems that face us as a society and face our species if it is to avoid what some have termed the sixth mass extinction, this one caused not by things like an asteroid, but by humankind, ourselves. Perhaps it can help us to look beyond the red alerts many have sounded about such symptoms of impending doom and their possible amelioration as war and climate change, environmental destruction, and mental illness, and consider human destructiveness from a more fundamental causal perspective. This is where a psychoanalysis more securely linked to biology as well as a biology more aware of and respectful of the unique contribution of psychoanalysis can enter the picture. If psychoanalysis can deepen its understanding of what is different about human destructiveness, it may have a uniquely important role to play in social enlightenment not only about causation, but about some of the difficult choices that humankind faces if fundamental change is to come about.

2

HOMO DESTRUDO

The manifestations of human destructiveness

Alongside our other remarkable distinguishing accomplishments, humans are more destructive than any other species.

The difference is qualitative, in depth, virulence, and extent, not just quantitative. In other species, the destruction of individual members appears to serve the constructive purpose of social group maintenance and species survival, but this does not appear to be true of humans.

It is natural to become habituated or inured to something so terrible as human destructiveness; something we seem to have no choice but to live with. That way we do not have to face our relative powerlessness, and in some instances bear feelings of guilt and powerlessness. Ironically, the defense of overlooking what we feel helpless to remediate may become a part of the destructiveness itself, an act of implicit acceptance. We court the peril of becoming a society in which hatred, violence, and less blatant forms of destructiveness like devastation of the environment become the norm; just the way things are. The adaptation of average citizens in Nazi Germany during the years of the Holocaust is a glaring example of such an adaptation; rationalized with such beliefs as it can't be that bad, or I was just following orders and doing what I was told, or in an extreme form of which we still encounter examples, it isn't really happening or it didn't happen at all. It is easy to look back on some of the more horrible events in our history and feel a combination of incomprehension, horror, and righteous indignation and wonder how people could have overlooked what was happening and not done anything about it, but there is a slippery slope that imperils us all. As I write this book, Vladimir Putin is in the process of making senseless war on Ukraine, using the most blatant vicious lies to justify his actions, and members of the US Republican party are supporting former President Trump's characterization of him as a

DOI: 10.4324/9781003442318-2

genius whose beliefs are always right, while he fulminates more outrageous delusional justifications such as that an election he clearly and decisively lost was "stolen" from him by a malignant cabal.

Denial of the unique scope and magnitude of human destructiveness unfortunately extends in more benign guises to those who have written about human social evolution for popular audiences and some who have theorized about it as well. Recent books aimed at a popular audience echo similar sentiments. The title of Steven Pinker's book *Enlightenment Now* (2018) reflects his optimistic conviction about humankind and its putatively glowing future. He views human nature through rose-colored glasses that seem blind to evidence of human destructiveness. He believes that humans have gradually tamed our presumed once-savage primate animal ancestry, and that as the result of stronger governments, education, cooperation among nations, increased prosperity, and increasing rights for women and minorities, war and violence are steadily declining and may eventually become obsolete so that presumably we will live happily and prosperously forever.

Yuval Noah Harari is another contemporary apostle of the doctrine of social Darwinism. Harari's book *Sapiens* (2018) has gained great popularity. His thesis is that advances in genetics and technology are leading inevitably to an ever more successful species, which will evolve in a humanoid or techno-human direction to become ever better.

Denial of the remarkable scope of human destructiveness is not the exclusive domain of popular writers. E. O. Wilson was the noted student of species' societies and creator of the discipline of Sociobiology whose groundbreaking work in sociobiology demonstrated that destructiveness in most animal species serves a constructive social and species purpose (outlined later in the book). In the latter part of his career, Wilson turned from the detailed study of insects and other non-human species to reflection about human social organization. The product of these later reflections is speculative, lacking the hands-on observational rigor characteristic of his field work with insects. In *The Social Conquest of Earth* (2012), he introduced the idea that human society is governed by what he called eusocial behavior. His hypothesis was modeled after the organization of ants, a species he considered an example of social success because of their seeming ability not only to survive but to thrive under a remarkable variety of conditions. According to Wilson, a successful or eusocial species is one in which the members have transcended individual selfishness and self-aggrandizement, and divide and share the task of population survival and growth among themselves so that not only the survival of a species, but its expansion, is more important than that of any of its individual members. Wilson refers to eusocial species as "hive-minded super-cooperators." In order to meet the definition of eusocial, or "truly social," animals must live in multigenerational communities, practice division of labor, and behave altruistically. He was seemingly unaware of the contradiction when in 2002 he estimated that if current rates of human-caused destruction of the biosphere continue, half of all extant species will be extinct by the turn of the next century.

Another more subtle way to minimize human destructiveness is to focus narrowly on one or more of its manifestations, like war, or destruction of the environment. Furthermore, not all of human destructiveness is self-evident. The context in which we interpret a given behavior, whether individual, social, or species, may determine how we understand it. Some of what in an individual and contemporary cultural context constitutes humankind's most impressive, civilized achievements turn out to be shockingly destructive when viewed in the broader context of the fate of the human species. And conversely, some individual and social acts that we automatically react to with a sense of horror as being destructive in their immediate social context might actually be constructive if viewed from the context of the long-term survival of our species. More about this later.

The phenomenology of human destructiveness

For simplicity of discussion, I have created categories of human destructiveness. Starting with the individual person, we humans are innately destructive to one another in ways that have no parallel in other species. Sociologists think of this as social deviance, and the origins of interest in the subject is generally attributed to Emile Durkheim (1895). Members of our species are always judging one another as bad, evil, wrong, inferior, and defective, and engaging in various forms and degrees of hostility, persecution, and even lethal attack on one another based on such perceptions, which may be based on race, ethnicity, color, religion, political belief, and even perceived psychopathology.

From a slightly different perspective, individual destructiveness includes such things as suicide; the psychoses that destroy lives both concretely and psychologically; drug addiction and society's current curse, fatal overdoses; criminal behavior; and less obviously, manifestations of basic failures of self-care that destroy individual lives and place burdens on society at large, many of which are subtle and easy to overlook.

The rampant abuse, neglect, and abandonment that characterize so much of our treatment of dependent children also constitute individual destructiveness. Such abuse is not limited to the egregious instances perpetually in the news about children in less developed countries, or even to the lurid tales of child abuse that fill the media day in and out. Much of it is more subtle; the kinds of rejection and hostility in parent-child relationships that fly under the radar of public attention because they occur within the isolated walls of family life. By comparison, parent-offspring relationships in most bird and animal societies that Wilson does not believe merit the designation "eusocial" meet the needs of the young during the comparatively brief period of postpartum dependence in a biologically determined way that is stereotypic for that species and lack the extremes of variability and pathology that characterize human child-rearing.

According to various statistics, more people are committing suicide than ever. The truth of this assertion is difficult to ascertain, as there is far less stigma attached to publicly acknowledging suicide as the cause of death than there was only a few decades ago, and some of the reflexive moral condemnation has been replaced by a sense of social responsibility and concern. In subsequent chapters, the distinction will be drawn between self-destructive behavior in species designed to regulate and maintain population homeostasis and such behavior that appears to serve no social purpose. Malignant forms of destructiveness are rarely if ever encountered in non-human species.

Psychosis is another self-destructive condition. In its extreme forms such as schizophrenia, it may culminate in suicide or homicide in response to delusional and hallucinatory mentation. Persons may kill themselves in response to delusions and what are called command hallucinations that "order" the person to engage in what from a realistic perspective are deadly activities, such as leaping off a tall building under the delusion one can fly or running in front of moving vehicles. Paranoid hallucinatory-delusional states can take such forms as commands from God, leading to the kinds of acts of social violence that regularly make newspaper headlines. The inability to take care of oneself may lead to homelessness or require hospitalization. However, in most instances, the self-destructiveness may not be so blatant as it takes the form of chronic disability that destroys individual life and is a drain on society.

Drug addiction, in its current form the epidemic of opiate-induced deaths, is a combination of individual and social destructiveness. Humans have always turned to mind-altering substances to alleviate pain and suffering, but they were not always so plentiful and easy to obtain. Our society has not come to grips with the fact that one of the reasons people turn to opioids is that the medical-pharmaceutical complex has successfully advertised that the first recourse for all human pain and difficulty is drugs. We teach our children this from an early age, and the result is people who turn to drugs to solve life's problems and then become psychologically and/or physically addicted. One of the medical establishment's major claims to power and prestige involves having a powerful therapeutic armamentarium of drugs, and mind-altering drugs have not only proliferated, but are routinely prescribed to alleviate mental as well as physical distress. Since the age of prohibition and bootleg manufacture and sale of alcohol, the criminal establishment has hopped on the bandwagon as well, producing an unholy alliance in which so-called civilized scientific advances have been used by medicine, the pharmaceutical industry, and the criminal enterprise, with the common goal of promoting drug use to the public. Their success is due in part to the fact that there are so many people whose immaturity or self-destructive tendencies make them receptive and prone to become habituated or addicted.

Social-cultural manifestations of destructiveness include homicide, terrorist acts, genocide, warfare, fanatical cult and religion-based acts of destruction, racial, ethnic, and class warfare, and extremes of hostility rationalized by differences ranging from gender to skin color to political and religious ideology. Individual and group acts of destruction toward others are woven into the fabric of human history and social change. As with so much of human destructiveness, so-called advances in technology facilitate or amplify such destructiveness. The single-shot muskets of second amendment days, laboriously crafted one at a time, that took great user skill and effort to harm a single person, have long since been replaced by automatic weapons designed to kill large numbers of people instantaneously and relatively effortlessly that are readily available to almost anyone and larger scale weapons that can decimate many persons at once. In the early fall of 2019, the *New York Times* summarized the violent summer just concluded, listing 26 mass shootings in 18 states of the United States, one after another, in the two months preceding Labor Day. The advances in weaponry and planes and missiles that can be used to transport and deliver them, and their ready availability to rogue individuals and nations goes way beyond guns. Bombs have become more sophisticated and relatively easy to manufacture and to deliver to a distant enemy, and in addition to the significant possibility of nuclear holocaust, we have new methods of destructive warfare; chemical, biological, and even internet hacking. Advances in communication afforded by the internet and social media encourage otherwise isolated destructive individuals to obtain the support and encouragement of a faux community to enact their hatred and get the peculiar notoriety that follows.

Genocide is a particularly virulent example of mass hatred and violence. Instances of genocide in the past century alone include the massacre of Turkish Armenians (1915–1918) resulting in one and one-half million deaths, Stalin's starvation of Ukrainians (1932–1933) causing seven million deaths, the Japanese "Rape of Nanking" (1937–1938) resulting in 300,000 deaths, the Nazi extermination of six million Jews, Gypsies, and miscellaneous others in the Holocaust, the 1992–1994 genocide of 200,000 Muslims in Bosnia-Herzegovina, the multiplicity of tribal genocides that continue to occur in Central Africa including South Sudan (Darfur), the Congo, Uganda under Idi Amin, and the Hutu extermination of the 800,000 Tutsi in Rwanda in 1994, and at this writing the large-scale extermination in Myanmar. Genocide is not just something that happens in other countries. Americans have been perpetrators, as well, including attempts to exterminate Native Americans and the life-threatening practice of slavery that in its historically attenuated unofficial form has continued as black people are perceived as threats to the established order.

Warfare is one of the most obvious manifestations of human destructiveness; one that with "advances" in technology is conducted on a larger and more devastating scale hitherto unimaginable. It is estimated that 37 million people died in WWI and 75 million people (3 percent of the 1940 population of the world) in WWII. Now that several countries have nuclear capabilities and the possibilities of chemical and biological warfare have become more real and sophisticated, such weapons can easily fall into the hands of immature belligerent leaders who might choose to use them, the worst may be yet to come.

Cult-related violence, often with religious or pseudo-religious rationalization, involves persons who have been unable to form a socially realistic secure sense of self. It involves subjugation of the separate identities of followers who become enthralled by their leader and the delusional web he spins. The leaders, all of whom seem to be men, are unable to exist without co-opting the identities of others to enact their agendas. One extreme example is the mass suicide of 918 people in Guyana in 1978 directed by Jim Jones, leader of the so-called "People's Temple." Cults are based on a binary of us against them mentality and promote violence toward outsiders who are perceived as destructive menaces. Examples include the murders committed by the disciples of Charles Manson in 1969 and the violent confrontation with authority by members of the Branch Davidian cult directed by David Koresh in Waco, Texas, in 1993. The Westboro Baptist Church in Topeka, Kansas, under the leadership of Fred Phelps, is a current example. It is organized around enactment of hatred toward persons of non-traditional gender orientation, veterans, and others who have been victims of catastrophes that the group believes are evil and need to be punished for violating God's will. Other than size and degree of alienation from society at large, it is difficult to draw a clear distinction between what constitutes cult destructiveness and destructiveness authored by political and religious regimes, for example, the Christian Crusades, the Catholic Inquisition in France and Spain, instances of Islamic Jihad, and the extermination of Jews by Hitler based on his rationalization of Aryan racial purity.

At this point, interjection of a few words about technology seems appropriate. The history of evolution of the second mental process is the history of transition from sociocentric to self-centric social organization that is described later in the book, and the simultaneous emergence of science and its practical application, technology. From the time this transition and the advent of science and the industrial revolution around 500 years ago until the present, it has been more difficult to distinguish whether the products of creativity and civilization are constructive, destructive, or Janus-faced in the sense of being one or the other depending on one's context and perspective. Technology has afforded humans the ability to fundamentally alter ourselves. It has produced forms of "intelligence" increasingly like what is human. It has produced various forms of social communication and related distant control unknown to previous generations. It enables us to fundamentally alter the environment and produce artificial environments with extremes of heat and cold, and atmospheric compositions, in which humans cannot survive, and equipped humans with artificial means to survive in them. It has produced forms of travel and transportation to places on earth and in space at distances and speeds hitherto unimaginable.

Finally, there are the things we believe from the perspective of preserving and enhancing individual human life and well-being are constructive, that from the perspective of preservation of our species may be leading to extinction of all species and destruction of our natural environment. History tells us that humans have never been primarily concerned with stewardship of the environment on which we depend, or limitation of the population to a size commensurate with available environmental resources. The problem has not been obvious so long as the resources seemed vast and unlimited, and the population remained both relatively constant and small enough not to produce global devastation. When the first European settlers invaded the American continent, it seemed like Eden in comparison with overcrowded Europe. Journals kept by early settlers who set about acquiring land and resources and eliminating its natural species in the process of "civilization" describe the abundance of wildlife of all kinds and the riches of the fertile environment. The now extinct passenger pigeons clouded the skies and buffaloes and other animal species the plains. Reduction in wildlife due to uncontrolled human predation and extremes of destruction of forests and plains in the process of building cities, roads, and farms has been so extreme that the west of today bears no resemblance to the Eden-like environment of only several hundred years ago. As the population continues to expand, depredations of the environment that once seemed inconsequential now take on more ominous meaning. For example, the tropical rainforest in Sumatra has been declared a World Heritage site and is nominally protected, but a recent undercover expedition there by a team directed by Matt Leggett, advisor for the Wildlife Conservation Society, discovered numerous unauthorized coffee plantations. Closer to home, the lobster industry in coastal New England is another example. Those Atlantic waters have been fished to the point where many species are vanishing, and control measures have been instituted in some places. An artificially created demand for lobster has become one of the hallmarks of the coastal New England vacation industry. All restaurants feature it. The waters are dotted with lobster traps. A lobstering license enables a single lobsterman (or woman) to maintain as many as 600 traps. In western United States lakes and rivers are drying up due to a combination of human-induced climate change and enhanced demand from cities and farms.

As human society evolved from sociocentric to its contemporary emphasis on the preservation and enhancement of the individual lives of each of its members, concurrent "progress" in medicine and sanitation has led to an explosive growth of the human population. Despite some of the shocking decimation of the human population already noted, there has been a fourfold increase in the past century and a threefold increase since 1950 alone. Several hundred years ago, child death was so commonplace that people often postponed naming children until they had survived the first several years. The average lifespan only a century ago was half of what it is today. The world consists of more and more humans, ravenous for space and for resources, entitled to resources and luxuries, and valuing of individual life over community survival. The number of automobiles in the United States has proliferated even more rapidly than the population. In 1900, the population was 76 million and there were 4,100 cars. By 1950, the population had doubled to 151 million and there were 26 million cars. In 2020, the population was 329 million and there were 287 million cars. This population explosion, coupled with the capacity to bring about drastic change engendered by science and technology since the Renaissance and industrial revolution, threatens irreversible exhaustion and destruction of the resources necessary for human life, and portends the potential for a lethal collision, not between earth and an asteroid, but between the human species and an earth destroyed and exhausted of resources.

The vast expansion of human population has created another destructive problem, the progressive accumulation of human waste products – trash, recycling, garbage, junk, waste, dumps – even things we think of more positively like monuments, memorials, archeological remains, and artifacts. The recent falling out of orbit of a 22-story Chinese space station focused attention on this problem myopically, raising questions about where it would land and whether the debris would harm humans and about increasing space clutter. The big question is the waste humankind is leaving behind, wherever we go. And perhaps the biggest question is that the problem is growing exponentially with the explosion of human population. The small helicopter deployed as part of the recent Mars landing accidentally discovered human pollution as far away as Mars in the form of debris jettisoned during the final stage of decoupling and landing.

Even though humans go to great lengths to keep waste products out of sight by dumping them in the ocean, creating dumps and landfills where people are unlikely to encounter them, and sanitation has helped in processing raw sewage and returning it to nature, our rivers and lakes and the sides of rural roads are increasingly littered with debris. Abandoned and exhausted mining sites are dumps for toxic materials. Possibly the worst example are areas forever polluted and off-limits to life as we know it by radioactive waste. Domestication of animals has produced the hitherto unheard-of problem of disposing of large accumulations of animal waste. Enormous floating islands of waste materials, much of them not biodegradable, pollute the oceans, to say nothing of what is out of sight and therefore out of mind beneath the surface.

Although it usually goes unremarked upon, when one walks in natural environments where there are few or no traces of human life, one rarely sees the remains of dead animals. Animal waste is also so rarely encountered that it is usually greeted not with disgust but with excitement, curiosity about the culprit, and discovery of an animal trail. In remarkable contrast, one cannot visit any human-inhabited part of the earth without finding cemeteries where remains of the dead are not only preserved in containers but memorialized with monuments.

Paradoxically, human destructiveness has become a popular riveting theme for the human imagination and some of its most remarkable cultural achievements, first through the oral tradition of storytelling and mythology, and in more recent times through written fiction. This is the subject of the next chapter.

3

HUMAN DESTRUCTIVENESS IN MYTHOLOGY AND FICTION

One of humankind's proudest civilized accomplishments has been to create riveting stories out of human destructiveness, a kind of phoenix arising from the ashes. The earliest stories took the form of what we now call mythology. Before written language, they were transmitted in the form of oral histories. Next, they became written accounts of events in which reality was not well differentiated from fantasies and epics. In more recent times they have taken the form of fictional written accounts; novels.

By approximately 3500 BC humans had developed the rudimentary abilities to communicate and to record and inscribe events to leave a historical trail, first in images, then in signs or ideograms. Around 2100 BC the advent of an alphabet enabled the first written traces of civilization and the recording of humankind's extraordinary preoccupation with destructiveness. From the perspective of reflective thought, we call the first records of human adventure and history mythology, as though they were records of fictional beliefs, when, in fact, they were as much historical records as are current histories, the difference being that events were viewed through the animistic anthropomorphic lens of primordial mentation, that from our current perspective mixed imagination with reality, whereas current histories are compiled from the reflective objectifying perspective of representational thought.

Carl Jung believed that mythology is an expression of universal symbolism that is expressed in dreaming and rooted in our biological nature. The thesis of this book is that both mythology and dreaming are expressions of a concrete primordial process that is concrete because it does not distinguish subjectivity and imagination from objectification of reality. Fiction, conscious fantasy, and history, in contrast, are accounts that are based on awareness that there is a distinction between external and internal worlds and that there

DOI: 10.4324/9781003442318-3

is separate content to be reflected upon. History is complex as there are two kinds of historians. One, writing from primordial mentation, is convinced that his or her account of the past is true and immutable, whereas the other, proceeding from reflective thought, is aware of the contextual subjective nature of any historical account and therefore its susceptibility to modification and revision. As for fiction, its creators know that however successful they may be in immersing the reader in their story, the mental productions are figments of imagination.

Mythology is not the exclusive province of so-called unsophisticated adults from antiquity or primitive tribes, however. It is an everyday creation of children at play and one in which adult caregivers sometimes knowingly participate, for example, the annual re-enactment of Santa Claus, or by purchasing toys that facilitate play, such as dolls and doll houses and toy guns. In the early developmental stages of transition between primordial mentation and reflective thought, small children often immerse themselves in words of creative imagination that to them are quite real. As adults some of us continue to engage in mythmaking. As we prefer to think of ourselves as sophisticated rational beings, we think of the product as what we believe in. The most obvious example of the mythology of everyday adult life is religious stories and rituals that are convictions about the world rather than symbolic expressions of faith and values. One person's religion is "true," whereas that of someone from another group is heresy. A litmus test for distinguishing symbol from myth is the question "Do you believe in God?"

The child immersed in his or her toy world, the dreamer, the religious believer, the cult follower, or zealot, all experience something like the person who is dreaming that seems quite real. It is only when the child grows up, or the dreamer awakens, reflects that there has been a dream, and laboriously translates the images and actions of the dream experience into language so it can be thought about, or the religious person or cult follower becomes disillusioned or is de-programmed that the product can be identified as fantasy.

With this introduction in mind, we turn to an overview of the mythology of individual and social destructiveness; toward ourselves and toward one another. The destructive understanding of the cycle of birth and death embodied in the class of myths known as Ouroboros, translated from a Greek word meaning "I eat tail food," is common to many different cultures over the eons. In this myth, depicted on the cover of the book, a serpent is devouring itself by the tail in a never-ending cycle. Ouroboros images have been found as early as ancient Egyptian funerary inscriptions from 1400 BC. They are also found in the Gnostic gospels and in such distant places as Hindu Vedic texts, Norse mythology, and meso-American cultures.

Warfare between the generations, or perhaps we might say within the family, parent versus child, is a common mythological theme. In Hindu

Vedas, the young generation of *devas* battle the older generation of *asuras*. In the Greek myth of the Titanomachy the Olympian gods defeat the older Titans. The Celtic gods defeat the older evil Fomorians. The Old Testament story of Moses and the Egyptians reflects this theme as well, as does the Greek myth of Oedipus in which the son actually kills his father. This play became the focus around which Freud constructed much of his theory of neurosis. The Mayans and Aztecs both practiced child sacrifice to propitiate their Gods. Bergmann (1992) writes of the role of child sacrifice in western religions. The Old Testament tells of God's instruction to Abraham to sacrifice Isaac, his only son. Around the same time, Sophocles wrote in *Electra* of how King Agamemnon had sacrificed his daughter Iphigenia to placate the gods at the beginning of the Trojan War. From the perspective that the animation of the cosmos reflects an absence of differentiation between the mythopoetic mind and the external world, the plethora of myths of an angry vengeful God who punishes humans for their sins also likely reflects the father imposing law and obedience on his rebellious children. Sibling rivalry is a theme in the book of Genesis, when the children of Adam and Eve compete for God's favor and Cain, the loser, slays his brother.

Oral aggression is a common feature of mythology. Ouroboros myths are one example. Hostility of mothers toward their children is another. Lamia, a woman of Greek myth, became a child-eating monster after her children were destroyed by Hera. In Zuni mythology Atahsaia, a giant monster, feeds on humans and fellow demons. A Pacific Northwest indigenous tribe known as Kwakwaka'wakw has a story of a man-eating giant who lives in a strange house with red smoke emanating from its roof. Shades of the death camps of WWII!

Many of the so-called fairy tales we tell our children are about giant monsters who devour children who disobey parental injunctions. "Fee fi fo fum, I smell the blood of an Englishman. Be he live or be he dead I'll grind his bones to make my bread" goes a rhyme that was first recorded in a pamphlet published by Thomas Nashe in 1596, along with the comment that it was already old. The witch seeks to devour Hansel after her alter ego, their stepmother, instructs their father to abandon him and his sister Gretel in the forest. The Brothers Grimm (1972) elaborated this tale, telling of how the wicked stepmother commanded their father to leave them in the forest to be devoured by animals as there was not enough food for all of them. In another of their tales, they tell how the enchantress traded the life of a daughter a woman was about to have for the Rapunzel, a green herb growing in her garden that the pregnant woman craved. And finally, in *Little Snow White*, a queen's envy of the beauty of the daughter she wished for leads to her attempt to destroy her.

One of the most common mythological themes, touched on in the Ouroboros image, has to do with the creation and destruction of humankind;

alpha and omega, the beginning and ending of the human world. Such myths are depicted on the oldest inscriptions in stone and their formal evolution from signs or ideograms to communicative language. The impulse to create such myths no doubt comes, in part, from natural cycles such as birth and death, light and dark, and the changing of the seasons. However, such myths also reflect an inner struggle that is deeply imbedded in our basic nature. In such myths, the world never seems to end entirely. One or two humans remain, or else there is a transformation or transcendence from the world as we know it to another plane of not quite human existence, exalted or degraded.

Mythology in which the end is not the end, and perhaps even a new beginning, reflects not only an inner struggle over destruction that is deeply imbedded in our basic nature, but perhaps a wish to deny the inevitability of death, as well. In 1961, Robert J. Lifton coined the concept of "totalism" to account for what he believes to be the universal human tendency to deny death. He describes the lengths to which humans go in order to do this, most particularly by the use of violence to abolish differences and create totalistic environments that confirm omnipotent beliefs, as was the case in Hitler's Nazi Germany (Lifton, 2017). In 2015, Solomon, Greenberg, and Pyszczynski elaborated on his idea of writing that much of "civilized" behavior is motivated by unconscious fear of death, leading to efforts to be immortal or superior that require the use of violence and conflict in order to achieve a sense of total power and omnipotent control. Mythologies such as the religious beliefs described next, that create totalistic belief societies, are one-way humans have tried to deny death. Another is mythologies in which the end is not really the end.

The major so-called Abrahamic religions – Judaism, Christianity, and Islam – have more or less common beliefs about the fate of humankind and its individual members. In these, there is an ultimate world-ending confrontation between good, as each of them defines it, and evil, and the possibility of individual transcendence from life as we know it to another plane or form of existence. The Torah predicts a cataclysmic end of days and describes *Sheol*, a kind of underworld. Later, Judaism, shortly before the advent of Christianity, developed the concept of a Messiah and a corporeal afterlife. In Christianity, the end of the world is Armageddon, *dies ire*. The concept of a second coming involves the return of the Messiah on Judgment Day to establish his kingdom on earth. The dead shall be raised, incorruptible. Those who lived according to the gospels can expect to go to an ethereal or non-corporeal realm where the light of God shall shine upon them. In Islamic tradition, after death the good go to a paradise and the evil are punished. In the ultimate apocalypse, fitna, Al-Malhama Al-Kubra, the good and the evil all go to separate realms and the human world as we know it no longer exists.

The end of the world is often depicted as climate catastrophe; a flood that covers earth and its inhabitations. One of the most common templates is about a wrathful or vengeful God who sends a flood to destroy all living creatures and a hero or heroic couple who are commanded to build a vessel that will take them and in some instances exemplars of other life forms to safety on a high mountain peak that floodwaters are unable to reach. Almost every culture has such a story, and they repeat over the millennia and regardless of geographic location. The fact that such myths are found in arid cultures as well as ones that are flood-prone suggests that they are not just historical accounts of floods and actual fluctuations in sea levels.

One of the earliest of such myths is the Babylonian *Epic of Gilgamesh*, written between 2000 and 1500 BC. The cruel despot Utnapishtim sends his friend, Enkidu, into the wilderness to seek, for his selfish gain, the secret of immortality supposedly learned by the person who survived the great flood.

The Hebrew Old Testament, written a millennium later, tells of a global flood that wipes out humanity and of the intervention of a god who selects a hero, Noah, to build an ark, do triage and assemble reproductive couples of all species, and raft them to safety on Mount Ararat. The Muslim Quran contains an almost identical story.

Hindu Vedic texts such as the sixth century BC Satapatha Brahmana and the Puranas tell the story of a great flood, Pralaya. The Matsya avatar of the Vishnu Shesha warns Manu, the first man of the impending flood, so that he can build a raft.

In Plato's *Timaeus*, about 360 BC, humans incite the wrath of Zeus because of their constant war-making, and he plans to unleash a flood upon them. Prometheus, who had created humans from clay, tells of the plan to Deucalion and advises him to build an ark to save himself and his wife. After nine days and nights, the water begins to recede and the Ark lands on Mount Parnassus.

In the Norse legend of Ragnarok, the world of titans emerges from an amorphous stew known as Muspell. There is a war among the giants leading to a literal blood bath from the wounds of Ymir when he is killed by Odin and his brothers Vili and Ve. There are different versions of the ending of this somewhat atypical flood story. In one, Bergelmir and his wife manage to cling to an object and are the sole survivors. In another the earth sinks into the sea and becomes Ginnungagap, a void. Ragnarok is sometimes translated as the twilight of the Gods and is thought to be the source of inspiration for Richard Wagner's Ring Cycle.

In Hawaiian mythology, Nu'u built an ark in order to escape a great flood. It eventually landed on Mauna Kea on the Big Island when the flood waters receded.

Mesoamerican mythology, both Mayan and Aztec, contains a number of different flood and survival accounts, in which humans are punished for neglecting the gods, for crimes such as cannibalism, or else the earth is simply too old and needs to be reborn. Most of the numerous Native American tribes also have flood and survival myths.

Numerous cultures, including Hindu, Buddhist, ancient Greek, Mayan, Hopi, and Mesopotamian, have a variant of the destruction and survival myth that does not involve flood, but depicts a cosmos repeatedly destroyed and reconstituted, like the seasons. For example, the four ages of the Hindu cosmos; the five races of the Greeks, who as the myth tells us live on after corporeal death as shades or souls in the underworld; and the six realms of rebirth in Buddhism.

These are creative depictions of destructiveness through mythopoesis, a concrete mental process of belief, to depiction through the lens of symbolism and creative imagination, the world of visual art and of fiction or novel. I should like to revisit the myth recorded in Genesis, the Abrahamic religion account of creation that to this day is believed by some to have been historical reality. Adam and Eve share with Prometheus in a somewhat earlier depiction of the punishment by the gods meted out to those who have the temerity to assume the knowledge, wisdom, and power that were intended to be the exclusive province of God. One of the central themes of this book is that sophisticated learning and knowledge accumulated after birth and transmitted to succeeding generations, which appears to be the exclusive province of species homo sapiens, has given us the power to control life and death itself and in so doing to subvert natural law or process hitherto common among species. The related capacity for reflective thought has gradually assumed precedence over primordial mentation and its associated belief systems, including religious ones. Hence, the Adam and Eve myth represents the struggle of religion to retain ascendance and control over the human mind and presages the growing capacity of civilization to control life and death.

Depiction of destructiveness in the arts and humanities

Visual art and novelistic fiction have emerged and evolved over the last several hundred years coincident with the emergence of self-centered cultures and reflective symbolic thinking. Such knowledge allows us to tell stories or paint pictures that we understand to be symbolic or fictional; figments of our imaginations rather than veridical truths about ourselves and the cosmos.

It would require a separate book to begin to list the artists who have created unforgettable paintings of human destruction and to depict even a fraction of their output. Many of the subjects of artists whose work we of western culture revere are religious in the Abrahamic tradition, and the earliest of these may have been intended as depictions of reality or the beliefs of their painters, much like cave art. A few of the many whose work is notable for its violent destructive themes include Bosch, Caravaggio, Caruso, Grunewald, Goya, Bruegel, Rubens, Blake, Monet, Picasso.

Finally, I turn to imagination in the form of fiction, the novel. Like the visual arts, the novel form is a relatively recent development, dating back about four centuries, which has flourished since the ascendance of reflective thought. Its early precursors such as Bunyan's *Pilgrim's Progress* depict the beliefs of their authors, much like the Gospels that comprise the Bible, and therefore reside in the gray area between myth and fiction. From its inception, violence and destructiveness have played a major role in fiction, and a Venn diagram including all novels that deal with human destructiveness would approximate the diagram including all novels. I have chosen to focus on a theme inspired by a recent development in human history, the emergence of sophisticated technology, a field that has advanced far faster than the maturity and judgment of those who have the power to use it. The astonishing proliferation of science-based technologies has inspired novels based on its misuse or disasters attendant to its use; nuclear, biological, and genetic. What follows is a summary of a few of the end of the world as we know it novels that depict destruction resulting from technology and its uses gone awry.

Alchemy was the precursor of modern science and technology. Mary Shelley was inspired by her visit to Frankenstein castle where alchemy experiments had been conducted, to write the grandfather of all destructive science novels, *Frankenstein, or the Modern Prometheus*, published in 1818. As is well known, it is the story of Victor Frankenstein, a young scientist whose experimentation creates a monster. It is not clear whether the book belongs on this list, because the technology involved, a kind of test-tube creation of humanoid life, was purely imaginative at the time of her writing, but she was a remarkable woman, so I opt to attribute to her a certain degree of prescience.

The more recent genre of techno-disaster novels appears to fall into two categories: social breakdown and world destruction, and genetic engineering of a new society of humanoid beings based on the equation of uniformity with perfection and superiority on the one hand, and variability, diversity, idiosyncrasy, and individuality with defectiveness and inferiority on the other – the kind of thing Robert J. Lifton has written about. The author of the godfather of such novels, Aldous Huxley, exemplifies the fantasy of construction of a new society, and a novel like Nevil Shute's *On the Beach* the fantasy of world's end.

In 1932, Aldous Huxley wrote *Brave New World*. He was remarkably prescient, writing about biological warfare and genetic engineering two decades before any other novelist turned for inspiration to such subjects. Henry Ford invented the first assembly line in 1913, when Huxley was a young and presumably impressionable adult. By the time he wrote the novel, Marxism was in its ascendency. Huxley was influenced by both. At a more personal level, he was also very interested in the use of flagellation, starvation, and drugs to create altered mental states that he called the antipodes of the mind and probably served as inspiration for his work.

In the book, after the "nine years war" in which much of humanity is destroyed by biological warfare – the use of anthrax – and presumably by the uncontrolled enactment of human destructiveness that caused it, some of the remaining leaders decide to create a new society in which people are free of passions, loves, and hates, and the personal and social ties emotions create, so they can be non-disruptive cogs in the social machine. Parenthetically, he is proposing regression to the old pre-enlightenment sociocentric culture in a new scienced-over guise. This "new" world is based on a religion in which Henry Ford is God (Ford = Lord). The bible of this society is an actual manual about the assembly line that was written by Ford. Time is measured BF and AF, and the iconic symbol is "the sign of the T." Creation of humanoid beings is moved from wastefully individualistic and destructively passionate sexual relationships to an assembly line modeled after mass production of the Model-T that produces hordes of identical humanoid beings in classes or castes, each designed to perform particular social functions efficiently. Batches are created from artificially fertilized eggs that produce identical multiples. The assembly process involves injecting embryos, infants, and young children with various substances, subjecting fetuses to unusual external conditions designed to condition them to respond to what they will encounter as adults, and once they become sentient, to further Pavlovian conditioning and nocturnal brainwashing. As adults, they consume large quantities of an ecstasy-inducing drug called Soma, much like we drink water, in order to insure they are on a perpetual blissful mental vacation, satisfied with their existence and non-protesting, as were the peasants in Feudal days prior to the advent of individualism. Creatures in this "brave new world" equate individuality with functional inefficiency, unhappiness, and social disruption, much as the Church of the first 1500 years AD equated it with evil. Relationships have no substance or permanence and are nothing more than transient sources of pleasure to drain off potentially disruptive emotions. The teachings of Ford and his bible are contrasted with an ancient moth-eaten copy of the complete works of Shakespeare, which is found and read with pleasure by a "savage" in a barbed wire-enclosed "reservation" where such primitive creatures, labeled as members of Native American tribes, are imprisoned. These savages use Peyote and Mescal to achieve states similar to those induced more efficiently by Soma.

About a quarter century elapsed from the creation of Huxley's prescient work until the appearance of more major novels devoted to the destructive perils of technology. WWII intervened, and perhaps the reality of the Nazi concept of a master race and the advent of the death camps and the use of medical science to experiment on and alter human beings, and the factory technologies and chemical gasses employed to eliminate socially undesirable types quickly and efficiently, came so close to such fiction as to paralyze creative imagination.

Ray Bradbury, a descendent of Mary Bradbury, who was convicted of witchcraft in the infamous Salem trials, published *Fahrenheit 451*, in 1953 at the height of the McCarthy era, another effort to crush knowledge and culture, specifically the banning and burning of "subversive" books and other manifestations of cultural creativity and free speech.

The novel is larger in scope than the destruction of individuality, thought, and creativity. It is a remarkably prescient description of the growing use of technology to brainwash people and render them passively narcotized receptacles. The protagonist, Guy Montag, is a fireman. The role of fireman has completely changed from one of preservation, putting out fires, to one of destruction, use of flamethrower-like devices to burn books that the mechanical hound has rooted out and burn those who have had the temerity to accumulate them. Montag and his wife Mildred live in a sterile house, three of whose four walls consist of television screens. The fourth will be purchased as soon as they have the money, leaving them totally surrounded by meaningless programs whose content includes intermittent opportunities for the viewer to articulate pre-scripted assent. Mildred spends her days with "seashells" in her ears broadcasting deafening music or the narratives of these programs; shades of the computer screen, virtual reality, and video games. When this degree of anesthesia is not sufficient, there are drugs or "amusements" that encourage the victims of this dehumanization to destructively vent their unhappiness and rage. The Chief fireman, Beatty, explains to Montag: "Why learn anything save pressing buttons, pulling switches...everything bang, boff, and wow ... Technology, mass exploitation...carried the trick...Thanks to them you can stay happy all the time... More cartoons in books. More pictures. The mind drinks less and less... We must all be alike...everyone made equal...then we are all happy, for there are no mountains to make them cower, to judge themselves against. So! A book is a loaded gun in the house next door" (excerpts from pp. 51–57).

Three years earlier (1950), Bradbury pursued the same theme of human destructiveness in *The Martian Chronicles*. The chronicles describe a succession of efforts to colonize Mars portrayed as an ancient civilization of wise, caring, cultured, creative people. Unfortunately, the inhabitants of earth bring with them the dissatisfactions and destructiveness that made them leave earth to begin with. They gradually destroy the ancient civilization and its peoples because its difference threatens them, and then gradually destroy themselves and their new land, while the earthlings left behind atomize the earth that remains.

The horrors of atomic devastation are referred to in Bradbury's novels but are not central to the narrative. Shortly thereafter, in 1957, Nevil Shute Norway, an aviation engineer for the British company Vickers who wrote novels as a sideline under the name Nevil Shute, published *On the Beach*.

This nuclear holocaust novel was made into an enormously successful movie two years later. This poignant story of love and death depicts the gradual extinction of life on earth as a consequence of the slow spread of lethal fallout from nuclear warfare from the northern to the southern hemisphere. The story centers around a small seaport community near Melbourne where submarine commander Gregory Peck and his crew dock their vessel in the course of fleeing the nuclear devastation. They set off on a reconnaissance mission to the northern hemisphere to determine whether there is any remaining life. As they realize their fate and lose hope, the story shifts to the agonizing decisions people need to make about whether and how to end their lives before radiation sickness ends them, accompanied in the movie version to the poignant strains of *Waltzing Matilda*.

Kurt Vonnegut continued the theme of nuclear holocaust with his 1963 novel *Cat's Cradle*, a bizarre satire about scientists and morality in which a Nobel Prize winner said to have been the "father of the atomic bomb" invents a deadly chemical called ice-nine, perhaps modeled after heavy water, an ingredient in nuclear reactors, while playing "cat's cradle." This substance is capable of instantly freezing everything to death once it comes in contact with real water, a kind of chain reaction. The scientist, who lacks a social conscience or moral compass, dies, leaving a bit of this unstable substance to each of his three children. The plot moves to a Caribbean Island run by a religious fanatic dictator. Through a series of Byzantine twists and turns, he commits suicide by swallowing ice-nine, and on the way to burial his frozen body falls into the sea and all life is frozen, leaving the narrator and a few other survivors.

Vonnegut published *Slaughterhouse-Five* in 1969. Focusing on themes of trauma and insanity in relation to the bombing of Dresden in WWII, and four years later, in 1973, Thomas Pynchon wrote his masterful raucous novel *Gravity's Rainbow* in response to Nazism, symbolized by the blitz of London with the V-2 rocket. The tone of the work of both these novelists is an unclassifiable combination of satire and dark humor. Tragedy and absurdity reflect the continuing effort of creative artists to come to terms with the destructive horrors of WWII.

The subject shifted to biological warfare in Michael Crichton's 1969 *Andromeda Strain*. A satellite sent into orbit in hopes of capturing microorganisms that might be used by the government as biological weapons is struck by a meteor and contaminated by a deadly microbe, which ironically becomes even more lethal when coupled with a nuclear explosion.

Stephen king's 1978 novel *The Stand* is a remarkably prescient piece of imagination that anticipates some of today's dominant social destructive concerns, including racial prejudice, the struggle between democracy with its imperfections and fascism that is more socially efficient at the expense of crushing individuality, government that perverts science to produce weapons of biological warfare, and social breakdown consequent to a plague. It also touches on dreaming and Jung's concept of a collective unconscious as a form of paranormal communication.

A lethal genetically engineered virus escapes a military laboratory and slowly kills most of the population, as society gradually breaks down. The government is more concerned with suppressing knowledge of what happened and denying that there is a problem for which it is culpable than it is with helping people and turns against the people who most need help in a kind of perverse alliance with the virus. A few people throughout the world who seem to have a natural immunity survive. Through a maze of death and uncivilized destruction, two groups of survivors gradually emerge and coalesce into opposing factions. The good people who have a pipeline to God through the corporeal mediation of an impoverished 108-year-old black woman congregate in Boulder, Colorado, and attempt to make a social contract and rebuild a civilized democratic society. The "evil" fanatics and cult followers congregate in Las Vegas – sin city – around a diabolical destructive dictator who binds his followers with a combination of threats and Faustian bargains, and the two factions prepare for a face-off that will determine the ultimate fate of humankind. Ironically, the book concludes with an inadvertent nuclear explosion that decimates the bad guys.

Of the numerous well-reviewed novels, to say nothing of numerous movies of this kind, the final one I have chosen to take note of is Margaret Atwood's 2003 novel *Oryx and Crake*. This is the story of one of the few human survivors in a post-apocalyptic world brought about by the remarkable advances in biology and genetics that ensued in the 70 years following *Brave New World*. The new society is run by an amoral scientific genius, dictator-guru named Crake, who uses genetic engineering to "father" in the laboratory a race of perfect inhuman-humanoid beings called Crakers, as well as other bizarre forms of hybrid animal life including pigoons and wolvogs. The new race of children is devoid of any trace of civilization, reminiscent of a benign version of William Golding's *Lord of the Flies*. In order to ensure the domination of this new race, Crake and his followers develop a pharmaceutical industry devoted to addicting human beings to a mind-altering drug called BlyssPluss that, unbeknownst to those who consume it, sterilizes them and causes the extinction of almost all of humanity, leaving but a few half-alive survivors. One of these is the narrator called Snowman, aka Jimmy, the son of one of the original perverse scientist-disciples of the guru-God Crake.

In conclusion, I turn briefly to *Moby Dick,* the iconic Great American Novel. It might be considered as a parable of the primordial mental process described in subsequent chapters, characterized by the absence of separation between self and other and the enactment of destructiveness based on the undifferentiated confusion of the perpetrator with the victim. In other words, Ahab is outraged that the whale has had the chutzpah to eat *him* (his leg) when the proper order of things ought to be that humans should consume whales, and he sets out with his primitive technological weapon to put the situation to rights. The novel depicts systematic human decimation of the whale species throughout the world for several centuries that threatens the species with extinction.

4

A HISTORY OF THE CONTRIBUTIONS AND LIMITATIONS OF PSYCHOANALYSIS AND OTHER DISCIPLINES TO THE UNDERSTANDING OF HUMAN DESTRUCTIVENESS

Freud created the discipline of psychoanalysis to study and treat individual human destructiveness and its vicissitudes. His belief that human destructiveness is innate, driven by biology, was echoed by Klein, who might be considered the other pillar of psychoanalytic theory until approximately WWII. Numerous psychological attachment theorists beginning at least as far back as Fairbairn, as well as Erich Fromm, whose work cannot be so easily categorized, have enhanced our understanding of the phenomenology of human destructiveness without considering its origins. Another way to say it is that they have implicitly adopted the assumption on which Freud's and Klein's understandings was based that all human destructiveness is based on a biological instinct to self-destruct.

Freud's theory of biological instinct and psychological drive

Freud proposed that all animal species share a common binary biological energy source, one of the poles of which is a death instinct, that he also described as a force inexorably attracting the organism into a state of entropy or dissolution, and the other a countervailing life force. In 1942, Eduardo Weiss gave the postulated destructive instinct the name "destrudo," which I have chosen as the subtitle of this book. Freud believed all animals, including humans, have a fundamental instinct to destroy, and that in humans, it exerts a force on the mental system that he called a drive. He explored the development and consequences of this drive, both separately and in conjunction with the life or libidinal instinct and its mental representative drive, in his economic and structural models, in the formation of character and neurotic symptomatology, and in the broader social structures that comprise civilization and its

DOI: 10.4324/9781003442318-4

limitations or discontents. He believed that the earliest humans were savages. He believed that in the course of our individual development (ontogeny) that recapitulates thousands of years of evolution of the human species (phylogeny), Thanatos, the death instinct, was mitigated though, not conquered by, Eros, the life instinct. Eros, through the mediation of its psychological drive representative, somehow motivated humans to develop the uniquely human manifestations of culture and civilization, and led individual humans to construct a complex mental apparatus or structure consisting of egos and superegos, defenses like repression and sublimation, and the capacity to make group alliances and identifications that take the form of law and government and mitigate but do not eliminate destructiveness. He recognized the paradox that the fuel for law and government is also a manifestation of collective violence toward the governed.

Freud articulated his ideas about destructiveness most clearly in the 1920 paper *Beyond the Pleasure Principle* and the 1930 paper *Civilization and its Discontents*. He wrote that "an instinct is an urge inherent in organic life to restore an earlier state of things which the organism has been obliged to abandon.... The ego instincts exercise pressure towards death" (1920, p. 44). In his 1930 paper, he describes various types of individual and social destructiveness as well as psychic efforts to counteract, oppose, and limit it including the neuroses. He describes character formations – sadism and masochism – that amalgamate Eros and the death instinct.

In the Freud-Einstein correspondence "Why war?" Freud concluded:

> The upshot of these observations, as bearing on the subject in hand, is that there is no likelihood of our being able to suppress humanity's aggressive tendencies. In some happy corners of the earth, they say, where nature brings forth abundantly whatever man desires, there flourish races whose lives go gently by, unknowing of aggression or constraint. This I can hardly credit; I would like further details about these happy folk.

Freud was not a cultural anthropologist, or he might have known that while there exist tribal cultures that are not destroying themselves, they have their share of destructiveness and can hardly be characterized as "happy." They simply employ aggression and destruction in different ways than we do; ways whose result is to regulate and perpetuate their social organization (Wilson, 1975; Robbins, 2011). But they are gradually being colonized and exterminated by the spread of "civilization," the supposedly enlightened force that might be killing us all.

Understanding Freud's rationale for the transformation of biological instinct into a mental process he called a drive has proven a daunting challenge for those who accept his ideas to explain. Virsida (2001), for example, has written a complex erudite explanation, but its highly abstract speculative nature and involvement of hypothetical psychic agencies and forces is beyond my comprehension.

Klein

Melanie Klein (1946) articulated a form of mental activity, the unintegrated and undifferentiated paranoid-schizoid position and its characteristic mental process called phantasy, which bears much resemblance to Freud's primary process, although she (and most of her followers) do not acknowledge the theoretical debt. As much as she tried to separate herself and her ideas from those of Freud, she and her major expositor, Hannah Segal (1993), believed that a biological instinct to destroy is the driving force of the paranoid-schizoid position. In her theory, the central problem of infancy involves efforts to survive in the face of rage and the urge to destroy that is present from birth. The initial mental state, which she called the paranoid-schizoid position, is characterized by splitting and projective identification designed to convert self-destruction into an attack on a misperceived external reality. Subsequent developments in response to maternal caring lead to a mental transformation to what she called the depressive position characterized as ambivalence, conflict, melancholia, and masochism.

The contemporary Kleinian view is well articulated by David Bell (2022) and based to a large extent on the writings of Money-Kyrle and Segal. Following on Freud's (1914 and the 1933 paper by Freud & Einstein), it is narrowly confined to intrapsychic explanations that might help to account for war. These include the paranoid-schizoid position (splitting and projective identification leading to social enactment of destructiveness) and the depressive position (melancholia; guilt and "moral masochism") that might result in its internalization. It includes the idea of "regression" in groups that might promote destructive enactment.

Like Freud, Bell assumes without further explanation the presence in humans of a psychological representation (the death drive and its vicissitudes) without concerning himself about how the leap from biology to psychological representation takes place or about the presence and reasons for a qualitative difference between humans and other species.

Erich Fromm

Eric Fromm (1973) is probably the most frequently cited psychoanalytic contributor to understanding human destructiveness since Freud. In *The Anatomy of Human Destructiveness*, he combines a little bit of everything: biology (genetic inheritance); sociology, cultural anthropology, and the history of civilization and society; and character and its formation in response to sociocultural and familial influences. His ideas are wide-ranging in scope, but he sacrificed breadth for detailed analysis of the linkage between each of these realms, the transitions between biology, psychology, sociology, and culture. He illustrates his ideas about character by analyzing the personalities of prominent destructive dictators.

In lieu of Freud's life and death instincts, Fromm writes of two polar opposite orientations, biophilia (life affirming) and necrophilia. He implies that individual orientations in one or the other direction are the result of a complex interaction among biology (genetic inheritance), culture and society, and familial environment. While he adopts a frustration-aggression perspective, he makes a clear distinction between defensive aggression, found in all species, and destructiveness that stems from necrophilia that he believes to be unique to humans.

Fromm emphasizes character and classifies destructive characters as sado-masochistic and necrophilous. He refers to the importance of the mother-infant relationship in the formation of character. When mother is cold and unloving during the phase of attachment and separation, the infant's orientation is narcissistic rather than biophilic.

One of his important observations is that the evolution of civilization itself has been in essence necrophilous, creating conflicting individual and social groupings, hierarchies and agendas that are exploitative, hence destructive, based on power and privilege. He notes that technology has been a part of this destructive force. Like Freud, he does not provide a map of the presumed transition between biological and psychological forces, nor does he map the uniquely human transition to social groupings that are innately destructive. In other words, he does not try to explain why humans have become more destructive than other species.

Frustration-aggression

The remaining psychoanalytic thinking about destructiveness subsequent to Freud's ideas about libidinal stage frustrations, Oedipus and castration, is not clearly attributable to a single individual but can be loosely grouped under the psychological frustration-aggression hypothesis, originally proposed in 1944 by Dollard et al. as a general behavioral principle. It has been noted that Fromm and others emphasized the critical distinction between aggression, which is a common non-destructive response to frustration in all species, and destruction, which Fromm and others, but not Freud, believe is unique to humans.

In 1973, the same year that Fromm's book was published, John Bowlby initiated the set of psychoanalytic ideas that has come to be known as attachment theory. Building upon object relations theory derived from Fairbairn, Winnicott, and others, he focused attention on the vital role of attachment and separation in the formation of a sense of self. I have written about the particular relevance of problems in the attachment-separation phase to destructiveness and psychosis, and provided an extensive bibliography elsewhere (2019). Of recent relevance to the role of biology in destructiveness, Panksepp and Biven (2012) write about the biological-somatic origins of affects that, including ones that are destructive, pathogenic infantile experience can transform into deeply rooted habitual tendencies toward rage, hatred, and destruction beyond the reach and transformative power of language and understanding. The model I propose shortly charts a pathway for understanding this transition from biology to learning.

Contributions from other disciplines

Scholars from a variety of other disciplines have explored and in some instances tried to integrate the subjects of uniqueness of human mind, human evolution, and human destructiveness. In reading the summaries that follow, it is important to keep in mind the questions of how humans evolved differently from other species, especially how homo sapiens has become so destructive and what the destructiveness portends.

From the perspective of ethology, Konrad Lorenz proposed a hypothesis about frustration and aggression that combines biology with population size. He believed that destructiveness is the consequence of hydraulic accumulation of instinctual aggressive tension in males, which may be triggered by frustration. In his well-known 1966 book *On Aggression*, he proposed that population expansion and overcrowding leads to build-up and eventual discharge of male territorial aggression. He does not discuss how and why the human population is expanding in a way that is atypical of other species. The aspect of his contribution that I elaborate subsequently is the cause and role of population expansion.

Richerson and Boyd (2006) proposed what they called the theory of gene-culture coevolution, or dual inheritance theory, that the biological and the social-cultural comprise a complex system with emergent properties. They give such examples as the evolution of the human brain and vocal apparatus, changes that, in turn, enable social communication and learning and in their estimation create phenotypes that favor survival, hence are selectively transmitted and perpetuated. However much they take important note of social and cultural factors, their understanding of the driving force of evolution is still basically biological. And the biology enabling verbal communication that they cite has by no means been as exclusively constructive as they imply. Destructive beliefs and ideas are communicated just as readily and effectively as constructive ones. They are cognizant of unusual human destructiveness, but they believe it can be sufficiently accounted for as an aberration within the context of E. O. Wilson's basic biological theory of species social structure that I elaborate in subsequent chapters that postulates destructiveness is a social and species regulatory mechanism, as when we aim for a target we don't always hit the mark. However, no other animal culture has "missed the mark" in such a major way that, to continue the figure of speech, the shooter shoots him or herself rather than the target. And in ignoring the extent and virulence of human destructiveness, they avoid confronting the possibility that this unique aspect of human beings might make us less fit to survive as a species, not more so.

A similar hypothesis is advanced by Henrich (2015). He proposes that cultural evolution makes humans unique and that its defining characteristic is social learning; the capacity to learn from one another. However, he operates within a Darwinian framework insofar as he believes this cultural learning is transmitted through genetic perpetuation of an adaptive phenotype, and in doing so, he also ignores destructiveness and makes the unwarranted assumption that social learning makes our species more likely to survive.

Most theorists of social-cultural evolution write from a social Darwinist context; a belief in progressive evolution of human socialization and culture, and ignore the dark side, human destructiveness. Robert Edgerton (1992), Robert Paul (2015), David Graeber and David Wengrow (2021), and the popular writer Elizabeth Kolbert (2014, 2021) are among the few exceptions.

Edgerton is refreshingly aware that whatever its other attributes, human culture is destructive. His book *Sick Societies* focuses on our ancestors and attempts to dispel the myth of the noble savage and the idyllic tribal society. But having made his point, he does not question its evolutionary origins, its seeming human uniqueness among species, and its long-term significance.

Robert Paul (2015) articulated a theory involving human destructiveness much like that of Lorenz. In *Mixed Messages*, he postulates that biological and cultural factors are independent factors in evolutionary conflict. The biological element is the male imperative to reproduce, which leads to violence and destructiveness. Culture, he believes, provides compensatory control and emphasizes community and cooperation. Culture progressively triumphs and accounts for what he considers the success of our species. It is mediated through symbol and language. He believes that, as did Wilson, humans are a socially superior, altruistic, cooperative species that is destined to continue to successfully solve the problems that arise. He does not attempt to explain the human difference of why and how culture has arisen in humans and not in other species or why the "male imperative" is not similarly operative in other species. Nor does he seem curious about the human difference, how culture arises. And Paul's belief in the mitigating forces of symbols is problematic. Calling the capacity for symbolism an unmitigated positive outcome of human evolution overlooks the fact that symbols do not have a fixed meaning and their use depends on person and context. When used symbolically, words such as black and white, Republican and Democrat, Socialist, vaccine, gun, and police can have positive or negative meaning and be used in ways that are culturally constructive or destructive.

David Graeber and David Wengrow (2021) and Elizabeth Kolbert (2014, 2021) write about destructiveness from a popular non-academic perspective. The deceased anthropologist David Graeber was a politically active anarchist, whose extreme views appear to have played a part in Yale's refusal to renew his contract as associate professor. His thesis is exactly opposite to that of Edgerton in that he claims that the proposition that we have evolved from savage destructive ancestry to increasingly complex forms of social organization, many of which are destructive, is incorrect. From his perspective as a dedicated anarchist, he believes humans have always been free to choose between more and less repressive forms of governance, and that these options have spawned the variety of social organizations throughout history, some more destructive than others. However, it seems likely that his predominant political bias has contaminated his theorizing. Whether or not this is the case, he does not ask how and why humans have evolved the capacity for free choice when other species have not.

Elizabeth Kolbert (2014, 2021) believes that human destructiveness is bringing about a sixth mass extinction not only of the human species but of all species. She does not incorporate the phenomenology into a broader understanding of human evolution.

Chapters 6 and 7 revisit the theory of evolution and examine its adequacy accounting for the human difference, especially human destructiveness. The next chapter describes the human difference in detail.

5

THE DIFFERENCE BETWEEN HUMANS AND OTHER PRIMATE SPECIES

Complex learning and the accumulation and intergenerational transmission of knowledge

A different approach to the problem of human destructiveness might begin with understanding the similarities and differences between human mind and behavior, human social organization and its function, and mind and social organization in other species, particularly our nearest primate kin. This approach will shed light on how human destructiveness differs from that of other species and why an assumption that all animate life is biologically programmed to self-destruct is incorrect.

Knowledge of our primate ancestors has been impeded by European colonial attitudes, mythological beliefs including religious attitudes, and the fact that most of us do not live in the jungle or around other large, natural animal habitats. With the move to "civilization" and away from a world where the species naturally mingled, our view of animals came to be divided into the domestic ones with which we are familiar, and "jungle" creatures of imagination, believed to be "wild" or even "savage." The gulf fed on long-standing religious beliefs that divided "man," made in the image of God, endowed with intelligence, language, moral reason, and soul, from so-called lower forms of life. The process of introducing the concept of primate intelligence to the average person is partly attributable to fiction. In 1912, Edgar Rice Burroughs published the first of his wildly popular *Tarzan* books, describing a fictional community of white British upper-class males and a tribe of apes. It is speculated that his work was stimulated by an event in 1868 in which a young British nobleman, William Milden, was shipwrecked off the coast of Africa and apparently lived for more than a decade with a tribe of apes.

In recent years, humans have returned to the study of other primates as explorers of a different kind; research by natural observation, a discipline almost synonymous with Jane Goodall. In her 1999 book *Reason for Hope*,

DOI: 10.4324/9781003442318-5

Goodall attributes much of her subsequent work to her childhood passion for the *Tarzan* books. She would climb up a tree to read the books and fell in love with Tarzan and was jealous of his paramour, also named Jane.

In recent decades, the pendulum of belief has begun to swing to the opposite extreme, the idea that other animals and a variety of non-animal species have personalities and think, feel, and communicate much as humans do. In 2017, for example, Franz de Waals published the bestselling book whose underlying assumption is laid out in unmistakable terms in its title: *Are we smart enough to know how smart animals are?* Perhaps the truth lies somewhere in between these polarities. Humans are unique, but that does not necessarily make us better, or superior – just different.

When we think of animal intelligence, we reference the creatures we keep in captivity, especially the domesticated animals who have become so dependent on humans that they no longer have natural groupings, societies, and habitats of their own. With the transition from hunter-gatherer societies to ones based on agriculture and farming, our most familiar animals became those we kept on our farms; now it is usually our domesticated pets. Most of us have either told or been subject to stories of "how smart my dog is."

Anecdotes about animal intelligence abound. A female chimp in her natural habitat in Zambia began to adorn herself by keeping a blade of grass in her ear, and others in her tribe imitated her and transmitted the behavior to the next generation. Amalia Bastos and her colleagues at the University of Auckland published a study (2021) in *Science Reports* of a Kea parrot they named Bruce, whose upper beak, which is essential for feather preening and cleaning, must have been destroyed when he was young. He had taught himself to hold a small stone between his tongue and lower beak in order to accomplish the task.

It is relatively recently that Jane Goodall "discovered" that chimps are caring, social creatures. She observed nuanced signaling interactions involving gesture and facial expression among members of chimp families and between community members, and understood them in terms of social organization based on emotional bonding and learning. Not long after she began her field work, major universities began to subsidize primate research. Chimp and bonobo researchers have employed spoken language, visual symbols, and use of computerized equipment to test primates and try to understand these processes in greater detail.

Students of non-human animal intelligence have divided research into sub-categories of self-awareness, use of language, emotional expressiveness, and relational attachment and bonding.

While examples abound of intelligence among dolphins, elephants, crows, parrots, and other creatures – most recently in the papers I read, an octopus – most of us think first about primate research. The best-known primate research has been done on language capability in primates that most closely resemble humans, chimps, and bonobos. Sue Savage-Rumbaugh, Allen and Beatrix Gardner, Francine Patterson (a student of the Gardners), and Herbert Terrace and associates are among those who have made notable efforts to teach primates to use language. From time to time, we read remarkable examples of their success.

To begin with the obvious, chimps in their natural habitat do not speak, write, or use signs or symbols, so investigating their language capabilities is challenging, and it is difficult to know in what context to interpret conclusions. Mind is the product of brain, the product of its capacities and its constraints. The brain of our closest animal ancestor, the chimpanzee, is a quarter the size of the human brain, whereas its average body weight is about three-quarters as much as that of humans. However, matters are not so simple as the critics of the idea that size matters have protested. Chihuahuas and several species of fish have bigger brains proportional to their body than humans. Sea lions have a larger frontal cortex than baboons. Lemurs have larger frontal cortex proportional to body weight than humans. Area 10 is one of the cortical areas of the frontal lobe involved in higher cognitive functions such as the undertaking of initiatives and the planning of future actions. It is larger in the human brain relative to the rest of the brain than it is in chimps. This suggests that the neural substrates supporting cognitive functions associated with this part of the cortex enlarged and became specialized during hominid evolution. In addition, other primates lack vocal apparatus and the Broca's cortex to control it that enables and supports human speech.

Nonetheless, there are remarkable examples of primates who have successfully been taught the rudiments of language, if its definition is limited to a system of functionally useful signs and signals and does not include representational thought and symbolism. Bonobos learn language best, and Kanzi is reputed to be a star among bonobos. Sue Savage-Rumbaugh and her team (2001) tried unsuccessfully to train Kanzi's adoptive mother to use a keyboard with signs that the computer vocalized as words when pressed, accompanied by presentation of the object or action they represent. Kanzi was an observer during his mother's educational failure. By age 6, which is approximately the time of full maturation for a bonobo, he had acquired a vocabulary of 200 words and was able to use them in instrumental ways combined with gestures or with other words. There are videos of Kanzi injecting his stuffed dog with a syringe in response to the command "Give the dog a shot." On another occasion, Savage-Rumbaugh used the computer to say, "Can you make the dog bite the snake?" Kanzi searched among a collection of objects until he found a toy dog and a toy snake, put the snake in the dog's mouth, and used his thumb and finger to close the dog's mouth over the snake. "Dog," for Kanzi, had a concrete meaning as a particular one of his toys. Kanzi was asked to identify 35 different items, and his success rate was 93 percent. On another occasion, he was asked over 400 questions and responded correctly to more than 70 percent. Kanzi and others who also learned the relationship between button pressing, vocalized words, objects, and actions were housed in a specially equipped dwelling that had button operated doors, a video with DVDs that could be selected with buttons, and a kitchen with a vending machine where they could get snacks. They developed their own taste preferences and, for example, particularly enjoyed DVDs starring primates interacting with humans, such as *Tarzan* films.

Washoe, a chimpanzee, was taught to sign by the Gardners. Washoe was able to transfer the sign for the adverb "more" that she had learned in relation to tickling to other activities she wished to repeat and to combine several signs in novel ways to make phrases to convey wishes. Washoe adopted an infant chimp named Loulis who was not trained by humans, but acquired more than 50 signs by watching its mother and other trained chimps. The investigators concluded that this instrumental language learning was spontaneously being transmitted from one generation to the next, analogous to the earliest stages of humans learning and use of language.

Francine Patterson, a student of the Gardners, set out to teach American Sign Language to a gorilla named Koko in 1972. She claimed Koko comprehended approximately 1,000 signs and 2,000 English words, but the comprehension was concrete, lacking in grammar and symbolic capacity. She likened Koko's development to that of a two- or three-year-old human child.

Herbert Terrace and his associates at the Central Washington University Chimp and Human Communication Institute (CHCI) were able to teach a family of chimps the use of sign language and the ability to converse with one another and their trainers by constructing meaningful sequences, one said to be seven signs in length. They appeared to communicate with one another about aspects of their lives together, such as signaling the wish to play games, like tickling and chasing. They were able to make simple category generalizations like small children do, for example, "dog" was used to designate all dog-like creatures (but not dog-like toys). One chimp referred to a watermelon as "drink fruit."

These observations demonstrate that although this kind of learning is not a natural part of chimp repertory, when captive in a human environment and exposed to opportunities as infants, they can learn more or less as human infants do, use the learning socially among themselves, and then "teach" their own infants and pass the knowledge on to subsequent generations. However, if these chimps were returned to their natural habitat where the learned knowledge was of no immediate instrumental value, it would soon be lost.

Franz de Waals emphasizes the contextual embeddedness or concreteness of animal learning. In his books, he gives numerous examples of birds and animals who make instrumental use of environmentally available objects as tools to achieve an anticipated goal that involves food provision. This is not the design and manufacture of sophisticated tools that characterize a member of homo sapiens who is not fettered by the imperative need to have dinner. He claims their intelligence is not sophisticated by human standards because what we call intelligence would be of no use in their world.

However, our ancestors once lived in "that world" and somehow moved beyond situational learning to satisfy less immediate visceral appetites to more complex "needs" like building spacecraft to explore the universe. One of de Waals's examples designed to illustrate the similarity between humans and chimps is that humans might have as much difficulty distinguishing chimp faces as chimps have distinguishing those of humans. However, once again he is illustrating a mind that is concrete, immediate, and stimulus bound. There was no immediate need for humans to have computers, fly in the sky, or visit the moon, but that did not prevent humans from developing the capacity to imagine such possibilities and inventing the means to actualize them.

Turning to self-awareness, another attribute of intelligence that has been tested in animals, in the 1970s Gordon Gallup devised a now widely copied experiment using a mirror as a research tool. He documented stages in animal development of self-awareness: social expressions, gestures, and sounds designed to elicit responses from another animal; physical inspection of the mirror to determine whether it is another animal; and finally, what he called the "mark test" in which the animal spontaneously touches a mark that has been made on its body that could only be visible with the aid of the mirror. This final action is believed to connote self-awareness. According to his criteria, dolphins and some whales, chimpanzees and some monkeys, elephants, magpies, and even ants possess this critical ability.

This is a clever experiment, but I believe that the conclusion that the self-awareness that is demonstrated is like that of adult humans is unjustified. It is more like that of the initial objectification of oneself human infants and small children copy from parent treatment of them but does not indicate the acquisition of thought and language reflective of a sense of self and other separateness or of an inner life distinct from external reality. In other words, the animal becomes aware of itself as an object, a "thing," not a separate cogitating subject like itself. I will return to this point throughout the book as I elaborate the hypothesis that mental dualism and the associated capacity to appreciate a world including others that is separate from oneself is a trait learned by humans as we mature. While human infants and other animals share a primordial mental process that enables survival and adaptation to immediate surroundings, reflective representational thought that is the substrate of creative thinking beyond the moment is the unique product of human development and learning.

Self-awareness and language development are related. The mirror test demonstrates that members of some other species, like human infants in the first couple years of life, are able to be aware of themselves as objects, but are not able to make the mental leap, signified by development of reflective representational thought, to view themselves as subjects. Infants can point to, name, and reach for objects of need and interest as chimps are able to do using keyboards or buttons labeled with signs. While chimps do not have language, the mirror test indicates that they can develop a similar sense of self-objectification. Small children can begin to use "I," denoting awareness of self as a separate being with an internal mind and things to think *about*, and soon thereafter become capable of using second- and third-person pronouns, indicating awareness other humans are separate selves, not just objects of interest; thus they have developed reflective thought, a mental activity not available to other animals.

Descartes's statement "I doubt, therefore I think, therefore I am" remains the best simple definition of the self-awareness characteristic of reflective representational thought. Noam Chomsky, long the Chair of the linguistics department at MIT as well as a prominent social activist, proposed that the distinguishing characteristic of language is reflective self-awareness, a concept that he called recursion. Steven Pinker, a vocal critic of claims by primate researchers that chimps have acquired language, states that recursion is a procedure that invokes an instance of itself: "all you need for recursion is an ability to embed a noun phrase within a noun phrase, or a clause within a clause" (1994). While Pinker is correct in inferring chimps lack this capacity, his and Chomsky's conclusion that "chimp-speak" or "infant-speak" is not language is based on an artificially limited definition of language.

Another claim made by those who maintain that the intelligence of other animals is like that of humans is based on the belief that they are capable of experiencing emotion, and that because some animals appear capable of specific recognition of one another and of caregivers after separations, they remember the way humans do. For example, a dolphin in an aquarium who had not seen another captive dolphin in 20 years was observed to be excited to see it when they were reunited. In his most recent book, *Mama's Last Hug*, Franz de Waals describes the deathbed reunion of an aged zoo chimpanzee and the primatologist Jan van Hooff, who had worked with her but had been absent from her life for many years. The listless dying chimp recognized him and reached out to touch him when he approached her. Similar anecdotes are often told about elephants. The reunions are accompanied by shows of what observers call emotion that are considered to be evidence of the capacity for memory. Naturalistic observers of primates including Jane Goodall and Alison Gopnik, and ethologists such as Carl Safina at Stony Brook, have observed chimps laughing, making deep attachments to kin, and suffering after their losses. This claim of similarity between humans and other primates, however, overlooks the critical distinction between affect, a somatic, physiologic, behavioral expression that, once again, is common to other primates and to human infants, and the awareness of specific emotions, which is an exclusively mature human attribute. And there is an important distinction between recognition of something or someone familiar that is enacted psychosomatically with gesture, facial expression, and vocalization, signifying an affective experience, and the presence of enduring memory, that depends on continuous mental representation of emotion and thought. Other than short-term searching behavior following loss, for example, there is no evidence the dolphin remembered its fellow or the chimp Dr. van Hooff. And no one would claim that these creatures "knew" the feeling or feelings they were having that corresponded with their behavior. Daniel Everett, the linguist and anthropologist whom I referred to earlier, studied the Piraha tribe whose exclusive reliance on primordial mentation I describe in Chapter 10. His work may help to clarify the distinction between constant representation that is indicative both of memory and anticipation and recognition of something psychosomatically familiar that has not achieved mental representational status. Everett observed that the tribespeople became fascinated with the float planes on which he and his family and others arrived and departed. For a short time after a plane arrived, many of them carved models of planes from wood, but the activity was transient as was any sense from their language that they retained memory of the event or that they anticipated a future arrival. When another plane arrived, they recognized it with excitement and appropriate language, but the recognition was bound to the stimulus, the sequence was repeated, and once again there was no indication that the event had been remembered and another coming anticipated.

The capacity for recognition on presentation of something that is familiar along with the expression of appropriate affect in the form of face-making, gesturing, and bodily sensations is very different from stable memory and awareness of the accompanying emotions, although the immediate behavioral consequences may appear to be the same. Human infants develop the sensory-perceptual capacity to recognize mother in contrast to other caregivers sometime late in the first year of life and to respond to her with facial expression, gesture, and vocalization, but there is no indication the infant is able to form and sustain an image of mother in her absence. When it is hungry and cries, it seems to need food rather than to want its mother. Such mental elements emerge later, as the language of pronoun representation reflects the movement from a concrete instrumental mind in which mother is equated with need satisfaction to one in which she is a remembered separate other person in the absence of felt need. It is not until well along in childhood that infants gradually stop expressing themselves by crying, gesticulating, and making other vocal sounds that sensitive adults can identify as expressions of emotions such as desire, fear, anger, pleasure, or despair, and with the help of adults around them begin to talk in the mental language of specific emotions about themselves and of desire for specific others. It is no accident that the primitive language of expletives is full of gastrointestinal, urogenital, and respiratory references that convey affects rather than in language expressive of specific emotions.

Mesoudi and Thornton (2018) named the issue in question cumulative cultural evolution (CCE), and they note instances such as I have cited in other primates and even in birds (navigation). They object to the idea of a qualitative difference between humans and other species. But they do not take into account either neoteny, the biological difference in maturation and environmental dependency that makes humans unique, or the acquisition of a second mental process, reflective thought, that results from it.

Popular science has rebounded from the widely held belief that other animals are wild in the sense of lacking intelligence and social cohesion to the opposite belief that they are capable of thought like humans, even if they lack the language with which to express it. It would be more accurate to conclude that the mental activity of other animals most closely resembles the mental activity of human infants and very small children and that there is a mental leap to the acquisition and predominant use of reflective representational thought that qualitatively distinguishes humans from other animals.

The basis for the distinction between humans and other animals begins with genetics and biology but is dependent on learning and the acquisition of knowledge. Human infants are extremely immature at birth in comparison to the young of other species. They require a lengthy period of dependency while they mature, whereas the young of other animal species are mature and capable of functioning independently at or soon after birth because their behavior is for the most part biologically programmed and stereotypic. Biologists call this distinguishing feature of our species neoteny. Stephen J. Gould (1977) noted the importance of neoteny in the development of complex social and cerebral behavior in the higher vertebrates. He says that the ability for an organism to delay its growth can lead to features that would support complex social and cerebral behaviors. For instance, rapid growth of the brain later in the development of humans could support complex cerebral functions. Gould claims that neoteny is the most important factor of human evolution.

An important consequence of the process of learning from caregivers that I reiterate throughout this book is that there is a broad variation in adult human personality compared to the relative uniformity of other adult primates. This variability, in turn, is transmitted intergenerationally from parents to children. As the saying goes, the child is father of the man.

The human brain is four times the size of the chimpanzee brain. The chimp brain is 40 percent of its adult size at birth and has reached full size of about 640 cubic centimeters by age seven. By around six, chimps are mostly mature and independent. Human babies are born when their brains are less than 30 percent of adult size so that the mature brain nearly quadruples after birth.

In addition to span of maturation, there are other differences between the human brain and that of other primates that may be relevant to the human ability to learn a second mental process. The human brain possesses speech centers that primates lack. Recent DNA studies (Pinson, 2022; Malgrange & Nguyen, 2022) have identified mutation of a gene known as TKT1 responsible for the enormous increase in frontal lobe size and complexity in particular, and brain size in general, that distinguishes Neanderthals and subsequently homo sapiens from other primates.

What these studies of biological mutation and evolution have yet to reveal is the reason for neoteny, the lengthy period of cerebral and behavioral maturation subsequent to birth that distinguishes homo sapiens from other primates, and that necessitations the dependency on and learning from parents that leads to the wide variety of human mental and personality variability. Chimpanzees are totally dependent on parenting until age 2, partially dependent until age 4 to 6 years. At that time, they meet the criteria for adulthood defined as the ability to forage and otherwise take care of themselves, to adapt to the local community, and the achievement of sexual maturity and the ability to reproduce.

And yet, chimps are late maturing compared to other animal species. Although there is no doubt that other animals learn from interactions with their environment, the balance of learned skill and behavior on the one hand and reflexive pre-wired biological response on the other is heavily weighted toward the biological and toward developments prior to birth, and the learning is mostly instrumental and immediately environmentally bound.

The long postpartum years of neurobiological and psychosocial maturation that set humans apart from other species require and enable a learning process and intergenerational transmission of knowledge that is unique in the animal kingdom. It creates a unique psychologically separate sense of self and a focus on individual actualization or self-determination. Other species that are more nearly biologically mature at birth live out a biologically preprogrammed adaptation to their environment and to one another that operates to maintain and equilibrate their social group (sociocentric).

The knowledge accumulated by transmission from human generation to generation that enables individual development and powers actualization of each person's unique abilities has produced the complexity and sophistication of human civilization and culture, which transcends biological survival and immediate community maintenance. Humans are able to learn from past experience and use the knowledge to create novel experiences in ways that transcend simple instrumental processes that satisfy immediate needs. This learning involves the capacity for conscious reflection and choice that enables us to expand our understanding and control over ourselves and the world around us. It enables us to transmit a significant amount of what has been learned to subsequent generations via education of our young during their period of immature dependency. But there is a dark side to this remarkable achievement. It also generates destructive clashes between social groups and creates learned destructiveness from disturbed interactions with caregivers. In other words, while biology is responsible for the basic difference between humans and other species, human evolution appears to be unique insofar as it is driven by learning and the acquisition and intergenerational transmission and growth of knowledge, as well. We humans have been to a significant extent freed from the imperative that biology is destiny, but the price we pay is that our knowledge also creates the possibility of a destiny that is more ominous.

6

THE THEORY OF EVOLUTION AND ITS LIMITATIONS COMPREHENDING THE HUMAN DIFFERENCE

The following chapters are devoted to understanding the difference between humankind and other species, which is largely based on the capacity for complex learning and the transmission of acquired knowledge from one generation to the next, from an evolutionary perspective. In order to understand the transition from biology to mind and the central importance of a psychoanalytic model of mind and its development, and how and why destructiveness has different origins and leads to different consequences in humans than in other species, it is necessary to revisit and consider modification of the theory of evolution. A review of the theory of evolution in this chapter will serve as background.

To begin with, the term "species" and the concept of evolution itself have become so deeply imbedded in common language use that most of us believe, without pausing to think about it, that we understand the meaning of these fundamental concepts.

Classification of species

Two hundred fifty years ago, Carl Linnaeus proposed the classification taxonomy of living things that is still used today. Though others less known preceded him, a century later, Charles Darwin turned the spotlight on the concepts of species and of evolution. The work of these two has generated much heat along with light; in an effort to clarify it in the century and half since Darwin's work, a new scientific discipline known as systematics has arisen to study the nature of biological diversity.

As is true with many important ideas that appear to arise simultaneously from many sources, it is an oversimplification to attribute the origin of the

DOI: 10.4324/9781003442318-6

study of diversity of living things to a single person. However, the work of the Swedish botanist Linnaeus is a useful place to begin. In 1735, during the age of enlightenment, he proposed an elaborate seven-level descriptive classification system that is still widely used, beginning with the most general distinctions and working down layer by layer to specifics. The distinction between human beings and other primates is made at level six, at which point the family of hominids is divided into four genera: pongo (orangutan), gorilla, pan, and homo (us). Some of these genera are further divided into species. The genus pan is divided into pan paniscus (the bonobo) and pan troglodyte (the chimpanzee). Of the genus homo, only sapiens exists today; Neanderthals are extinct, and erectus is presumed to be our ancestor. The members of genus homo were distinguished by large cranial capacity, erect posture and bipedal gait, opposable thumbs, and the ability to make sophisticated standardized tools.

A century after Linnaeus, in 1859, Darwin wrote *On the Origin of Species*. The hierarchical concept of evolution through natural selection is credited to him although it was apparently discovered more or less concurrently and independently by Alfred Russel Wallace. The theory is that survival and transmission of the most adaptive mutations accounts for why species differ from one another and how they develop or evolve from common ancestry. Remarkably, Darwin never clearly defined what constitutes a species. He distinguished two groups of living things, species and varieties. In *Origins*, he makes the somewhat ambiguous distinction:

> Hereafter we shall be compelled to acknowledge that the only distinction between species and well-marked varieties is, that the latter are known, or believed, to be connected at the present day [to existing species] by intermediate gradations, whereas species were formerly thus connected.
>
> *(1859, p. 485, bracketed comment mine)*

In *The Descent of Man* (1871), he writes:

> Practically, when a naturalist can unite two forms together by others having intermediate characters, he treats the one as a variety of the other, ranking the most common, but sometimes the one first described, as the species, and the other as the variety. But cases of great difficulty sometimes occur in deciding whether or not to rank one form as a variety of another, even when they are closely connected by intermediate links; nor will the commonly assumed hybrid nature of the intermediate links always remove the difficulty.
>
> *(pp. 214–215)*

He appears to be stating that species lack the obvious progression that would be suggested by intermediate forms, which he called varieties, even though they presumably evolved from varieties. By this criterion, sapiens and Neanderthal are varieties of genus homo, but only sapiens has survived as a species.

That his hypothesis of evolution by natural biological selection applied to humans as well is made clear in Chapter 5 of *Descent* when he states his belief that the mental differences that distinguish humans from other animals have unequivocal survival value.

Some consider Jean-Baptiste (Pierre Antoine) de Monet, the Chevalier de Lamarck, to be responsible for the study of evolution of species rather than Darwin. In 1809, almost half a century before Darwin, he wrote *Philosophie Zoologique*, a treatise in which he coined the term *biology* and proposed the first scientific theory of evolution, that all species are descendants of common simple forms. He encountered fierce criticism, however, including from Darwin half a century later, who called his ideas "nonsense" while ironically incorporating the idea of species descent into his own theory. In 1902, the German biologist Ernst Haeckel distinguished between the common descent aspect of evolution which he attributed to Lamarck and the natural selection aspect which he attributed to Darwin. Lamarck's belief that acquired characteristics could be transmitted has been ridiculed, but apparently his ideas were misunderstood because of poor translation of his books. The idea that the transmission is direct, and that the characteristics in question might be ones developed by use during life, is usually ridiculed by illustrating it with the example that giraffes grow longer necks by exercise in order to get the choicest food or the strength of the blacksmith might be inherited. He actually wrote: "For, whatever the environment may do, it does not invoke any direct modification in the shape and organization of animals." At the same time that Lamarck is usually dismissed out of hand, his ideas have survived in an active controversy among evolutionary biologists within the field of epigenetics.

The term epigenetics was introduced by embryologist Conrad Waddington in 1957. It designates the complex of developmental processes between the genotype and phenotype; what is called the epigenome. He maintained that our life habits and experiences modify genetic material, and do not just contribute to the survival of organisms and selective propagation of their genes. Critics of epigenetics point out that the kinds of changes that are referred to consist of environmental and behavioral habit factors that tend to degrade the organism, hence the changes would not be adaptive and would probably lead to species deterioration rather than to evolution defined as survival. That critique would certainly seem to apply to human destructiveness.

Early objections to Darwin's theory came from creationists; those who came to science through a Christian religious background and who were torn between scientific objectification and the Biblical teaching that humans are made by God in his image and hence are qualitatively different from and superior to savage animal creatures. Richard Owen (1860) proposed a quasi-religious definition of species that continues to have supporters today, based on breeding purity. In other words, if two animals could not mate and produce young, then they were of different species. By this criterion, chimps and humans are not members of the same species. Darwin disagreed with the proposition that hybrid sterility is an adequate definition of speciation. What these critics failed to take into account is that the human species is different but looking to religion to comprehend the difference is a form of barking up the wrong tree.

Ernst Mayr and Theodosius Dobzhansky, two of the most influential twentieth-century contributors to the field of systematics, also objected to Darwin's theory that species are continuous with lower-level forms and have evolved by natural selection. They proposed instead that species are populations that have become reproductively inbred because of geographic isolation from one another.

Gregor Mendel's nineteenth-century discovery of genetics through his research with plants, propelled by subsequent advances in biology and the development of sophisticated mathematical models, has fundamentally altered the dialogue about species and has served to direct the study of evolution toward the understanding of microscopic forms, genes, and DNA. In the last century, distinct fields including population genetics, evolutionary biology, epigenetics, and molecular genetics have arisen along with efforts to integrate them. They share a common view of evolution based on biology and propagation of the genes whose phenotypes have proven most adaptive and have led to lively debates over such things as the relative importance of genetic drift, gradual changes in a population related to the random disappearance of particular genes, and alteration of genes based on life experience that has led to selective propagation of their phenotypes.

In the late nineteenth century, social scientists began efforts to move the dial in the other direction but the predominant microbiological focus has not changed. Richard Dawkins (1976) wrote about genes as the self-propagating living structures, and described how they act indirectly, through their phenotypes, or somatic embodiments in his bestselling book *The Selfish Gene*; he described how natural selection modifies genes by favoring the survival and propagation of some phenotypes and not others. As Herbert Gintis (2011) points out, transmission via selection of phenotypes is epigenetic, not genetic. That is, it is the study of the expression of genes, not the genes themselves.

In efforts to relate the microscopic world of molecular genetics to the macroscopic world of living animals, the Smithsonian Human Evolution Project has studied the genetic similarities and differences among members of the genera pan and homo. The variation in DNA among humans is but

0.1 percent. Between humans on the one hand and chimps and bonobos on the other, it is but 1.2 percent. The difference between chimps, bonobos, and humans considered as a group, and gorillas, is 1.6 percent. In other words, there is a 98.5 percent similarity in DNA amongst us. DNA, however, is a building block, and it can be present in different quantities and different configurations in the genome. When complexities such as this are taken into account, there appears to be a 4–5 percent difference between humans and chimpanzees.

7

REVISING THE THEORY OF EVOLUTION TO ACCOUNT FOR THE HUMAN DIFFERENCE

The mental capacity of chimps and bonobos is much like that of human infants and very young children. If removed from their natural environment and held captive in a laboratory where they are taught by human researchers, they can learn primitive sign language. However, these skills are not natural to them. If they raise their young in the research laboratory setting where such skills are useful, they can teach them to succeeding generations. The limitation on transmission of acquired knowledge and skill is based on the capacity of brain as well as speech centers and vocal apparatus. These things impose a ceiling on the ability to move beyond biologically determined primordial mental activity that enables survival of the individual and maintenance of homeostasis of the group in their natural habitat.

Chapter 4 describes the contributions of psychoanalysis and other disciplines to understanding the human difference, especially as it relates to destructiveness; the mental and social developments that set homo sapiens apart from other species. It includes the unsatisfactory efforts made by numerous anthropologists and others to modify the theory of evolution to account for it. In 1895, James Baldwin, a Princeton psychologist, was perhaps the first to express concern that evolution theory did not take into account mental and social factors. A century elapsed between that time and commencement of a more serious discussion of the human difference by Donald Campbell (Hayes & Hull, 2001), originator of what is known as realistic conflict theory. The work of others including Richerson and Boyd, Joseph Henrich, Robert Edgerton, E. O. Wilson, Elizabeth Kolbert, and David Graeber was summarized and critiqued in Chapter 4, which focused on human destructiveness. None have adequately accounted for whether and how a biological theory of evolution can account for the psychosocial human difference from other

DOI: 10.4324/9781003442318-7

species, or whether the theory of evolution needs modification to include independent psychosocial as well as biological causation. These last two statements may appear to be contradictory, but they are not. A different understanding of the biology of evolution can enable us to understand how learning and complex acquisition of knowledge acts as an independent evolutionary force and accounts for the human difference.

There is a biological difference between homo sapiens and other species whose influence on evolution has not been appreciated that does enable us to take these things into account. The phenomenon known as neoteny, or extended postnatal immaturity (Gould, 1977), has a unique effect on human development and species evolution. The consequences of neoteny are a prolonged enforced dependency on caregivers that enables and requires social learning and the acquisition of sophisticated knowledge, including the development of a second mental process, reflective thought. As a result, extensive learning occurs in the process of each individual person's development, and this learning leads to knowledge that can be transmitted and expanded from generation to generation. The theory of evolution that is generally accepted attributes change exclusively to the biology of genetic mutation and of perpetuation of phenotypes most favorable to survival. It needs to be modified to include the possibility that complex learned knowledge, transmitted from one generation to the next, can act as an evolutionary force independent of biology. The content of this knowledge includes not only those elements that we consider civilized, creative, and culturally sophisticated, but also the unique attributes of human destructiveness. This constitutes the human difference.

The forces of change that stem from learning and the acquisition, accumulation, and intergenerational transmission of knowledge have given rise to culture and civilization, but also to an extent, intensity and virulence of human destructiveness that has no parallel among other species and is not easily accounted for by a biological reductive survival-adaptive theory of evolution. Human destructiveness seems to go well beyond what E. O. Wilson envisioned as the forces that act to maintain and stabilize social organization in other species that are described in Chapter 10.

The problem of human destructiveness is further complicated by the fact that it is not always obvious. Chapters 2, 12, 16, and 17 in particular elaborate aspects of civilization that in the context of actualization of the potential of individuals are constructive but in a broader social and evolutionary context are not. Perhaps the most significant of these seeming signs of progress is the flourishing of humankind. The population is expanding at an astonishing exponential rate. Wilson related humans to ants in this regard and interpreted population expansion as indicative of species success, presumably because it does not have the actual and potentially devastating consequences that the remarkable and very recent growth of the human population portends.

Others understand it as a "not to worry" problem for which our remarkable social capacities will find a solution. In Chapter 17, the possible consequences of an unchecked expansion of population on human society, on other species, and on the environment are examined in detail.

Scientists have concluded that in the course of life on earth, more than 99 percent of species have become extinct. In most instances of species extinction, the destruction was not related to behavioral factors related to the genetic makeup of members of the species but was the result of extraneous factors – natural disasters and environmental changes beyond the control of species' ability to adapt, such that the environment became inimical to survival. It is generally believed that over the course of life on earth, there have been five mass extinctions, each caused by disruption of elements of the environment vital to sustaining life – atmosphere, water, plant life – and each resulting from a natural disaster such as volcanic eruption or asteroid collision. In 1992, Michael Novacek, curator at the Museum of Natural History, proposed that we are now in the midst of a sixth mass extinction, this one different from all those preceding insofar as the external cause is not a natural disaster but is the rogue behavior of the human species itself, including a combination of direct destruction of other species, destruction of the environment on which they depend, and expansion of the human population to a point that is environmentally unsustainable for life.

Popularization of the concept of a sixth mass extinction caused by humankind is generally attributable to Elizabeth Kolbert (2014). Kolbert's focus is on technology. In her 2021 book *The White Sky*, whose title is taken from a likely consequence of one of the ecological "fixes" scientists are currently contemplating, she describes the inexorable progression (or regression?) of destructiveness caused by what might be captioned by the saying that the cure is worse than the disease. Human "fixes" have made things worse and often created new and unforeseen problems. And the beat goes on!

The biology of neoteny and the related psychology of learned knowledge provide an understanding of the uniqueness of homo sapiens. Complex human learning and the intergenerational transmission and growth of knowledge distinguish humans from all other species. The remarkable creative achievements of culture and civilization are well known. This book has undertaken to review, critique, and expand psychoanalytic understanding of human destructiveness originating with Freud's contributions. Its focus is on the implications of the destructive aspect of the human difference for us as individuals, for human society, and for the evolution of our species. There seem to be two possible consequences for the human species, one more optimistic than the other. The first is that however remarkable the difference between us and other primates may seem, the human species still conforms to the principles that govern life and death of other species that Wilson outlined that are explained in Chapter 10, in which destructiveness serves a social regulatory function. This possibility poses major problems for humans who value individual life and yet have serious concerns about the future of our species and our planet. We humans would need to take drastic measures, some of which would be basically at odds to prevailing values and mores, if our species is to have a chance to survive. These problems are explored in the concluding chapters.

A second possibility is that the human difference fits neatly into the biological theory of evolution of species and homo sapiens as an instance of a fatal mutation or combination of mutations. In that case, neoteny and its consequences will not be compatible with long-term species survival. Considering the vast expanse of evolutionary time rather than the brief period that homo sapiens has walked the earth, perhaps our species is but a brief candle, an evolutionary mistake.

As background for the discussion to come, it will be useful to describe the mental process that sets humans apart from other species that is the consequences of the biology of neoteny and its results, the long period of postnatal learning from caregivers, and its development in the course of maturation.

8

THE UNIQUE NATURE OF HUMAN MIND

Reflective representational thought

Although humans share a common primordial mental process with other animals, there is a fundamental difference. Human mind and behavior are qualitatively unique because of our acquisition of a second mental process, reflective representational thought. As a result, we can acquire complex knowledge and transmit it to subsequent generations, where over time it can accumulate into a complexity of culture and civilization (and destructiveness) unimaginable in other species. This is the consequence of our prolonged period of extrauterine immaturity and dependency on and learning from caregivers. This chapter describes the dual nature of mind that is unique to humans, and the one that follows describes the development of the second process that sets us apart from our common animal origins.

History of the conception of human mind as a dual structure

Freud may have been the first to propose that a dual mental process is characteristic of humans. In 1900, he articulated the concept of a primary process, derived from his study of dreaming, that ontologically precedes the development of what he called secondary process thought. He believed the primary process is the mentation of infants and the secondary process of adults, and that developmental problems sometimes lead to kinds of contamination of the latter by the former. Perhaps because his understanding of the primary process came from the study of dreams, and we dream when we are asleep, and because the primary process lacks the aspect of self-awareness, he believed the process is unconscious, whereas it is simply conscious in a different way, as is dreaming, a way we share with other intelligent creatures that lack the capacity to reflect on the contents of their minds. Freud's fateful decision has

DOI: 10.4324/9781003442318-8

lent an air of mystery and opacity to this basic mental activity and has led to other confusion, such as the mistaken belief that infants are not conscious.

In fact, this primordial form of mentation is a different form of consciousness than reflective thought, which implies the Cartesian capacity to introspect, and the awareness that there is a subjective "I" and a separate objective "thou." While there appears to be an "I" in dreams, in the sense of an experiencing subject, and there are "others," as well, the "I" is not a reflective "I" but an illusion of participation in a drama that feels real. And the "thou" is not another "real" person with whom the dreamer is interacting, as in waking life, but a depiction of an aspect of the dreamer's mind.

Freud discovered the primary process through waking thoughtful contemplation of the nature and significance of his own dreams. He described the characteristics of the primary process as displacement, condensation, and absence of contradiction. The mental contents or ideas that are separate and distinct from one another in waking life, expressed in reflective thought, that he called the secondary process, are not differentiated from one another and contents that take the form of thoughts or ideas in waking life are expressed as an enactment or dramatization in the primary process. The primary process creates a sensory-perceptual identity; a false sense of reality unfolding that, as he noted, resembles hallucination and delusion in waking life. Wishes and other repudiated ideas are experienced as reality. For example, Donald Trump does not say "I wish I had won the election," he says "I won the election and it was stolen from me."

The major feature of the primary process is absence of differentiation between mind and world. The primary process creates a narrative linked not by elements of logic, consensual reality, and sense of time, but by predominant affects, moods, or feeling states. Things are put together that would not ordinarily happen in real life. As there is no reflective thought and no realistic distinction between mental elements, the dream itself is concrete, not symbolic. We can create symbols, analogies, and other linguistic characteristics distinguishing words from things out of our dreams once we awaken and emerge from the dream state, and much of Freud's therapeutic method depends on doing so, but this requires that we recognize we have had a dream, laboriously translate the imagery and actions into a thoughtful narrative about which we can reflect, and then look for symbolic meaning in that context.

Others have followed Freud in proposing that human mind works in two qualitatively different ways, most notably the cultural anthropologist Lucien Lévy-Bruhl (1923, 1928, 1935), Julian Jaynes (1976), and more recently (2011) Daniel Kahneman. From the perspective of cognitive developmental psychology, Jean Piaget (1936,1952) developed a four-stage model, the first three stages of which (sensorimotor, preoperational, and concrete operational) bear some resemblance to primordial mental activity.

The work of Piaget and Kahneman is of limited relevance to this discussion as it is focused on cognition and excludes the body and our affects, that as our minds mature become our emotions, which are the origins and drivers of our minds. Piaget's model of cognitive development is a sophisticated description of the earliest sensorimotor phase in which mentation is immediate, concrete, and enactive, but his model has no place for the body and its affective expressions. A few years ago, Kahneman wrote the popular book *Thinking Fast and Slow*. His focus is mostly on practical functional applications of the cognitive process he describes. The similarity to primordial mentation is what he calls fast thinking. It is reflexive and forms beliefs or intuitions that are useful under certain situations that require rapid response but are impediments in others where deliberate, contemplative, logical thinking and evidence gathering is called for. Bonobos are quicker than older human children in solving some simple problems because they are not burdened with having to think too much about what they are doing.

About a quarter century after Freud's discovery of the primary process, the cultural anthropologist Lucien Lévy-Bruhl wrote a series of books (1923, 1928, 1935) describing the mental activity of tribal people he had observed, that he called primitive because it is not governed by logic, as is the working of the "modern" or European mind of Lévy-Bruhl and his fellow anthropologists. He described the inability of primitive mind to differentiate the supernatural from reality and to recognize and deal with contradictions. But his terminology suggests that he believed he was describing an inferior race, not a different form of mentation that is socially and functionally adaptive under the circumstances in which it occurs. What others call anthropomorphizing or animation of the world, he referred to as the process of "mystical participation." Lévy-Bruhl did believe that residues of these "prelogical" elements continue to exist in a mature mind along with "logical" ones, or to say it differently, that the two processes are to be found in the ordinary functioning of an adult mind. He believed that except for these remnants, mind had evolved over the ages from its original tribal beginnings to European sophistication.

It is important to separate Lévy-Bruhl's basic ideas from the cultural bias or judgmentalism prevalent at the time he formulated them. Even in this more enlightened era, most of us share the prejudice that logic, science, and technology make us superior, not just different. We tend to believe that the term "mythology" is a perfectly acceptable name for products of the other process, drawing an imaginary line between the belief that we know better, and they didn't know any better, heedless of the fact that the other process plays a significant role in our contemporary life as well, and when it does, we do not call it mythology. Chapter 3 describes the nature of mythology, its persistence in some aspects of contemporary culture, principally religion and other passionately held beliefs that are not subject to "reason" and reflective thought.

Three-quarters of a century after Freud's discovery of the primary process, Julian Jaynes published the evolutionary hypothesis about mind and brain he called bicameralism.

The brain of homo sapiens, he believed, originated 3,000 years ago as a bicameral structure whose right and left hemispheres housed different functions and were not connected. He believed that the cerebral hemispheres function qualitatively differently, the left responsible for reflection and self-regulation and the right producing emotion and action, and that mature functioning requires their integration through the interconnecting cerebral commissure connecting them. He believed that early homo sapiens lacked a cerebral commissure, and hence, early societies and cultures were evanescent because they could not control and regulate destructive action.

What he called right brain behavior closely resembles Freud's description of the primary process and what I call primordial mentation. He described what he believed to be an unconscious process involving loss of the "analog I" or the sense of one's separate self and one's mind; the dissolution of mind-space, by which he means the capacity to introspect or reflect on one's mind; and the absence of what he called narratization; the ability to construct a story about oneself rather than live in the story. Along with Descartes and Freud, he defined consciousness as self-awareness, reflection, and introspection, so he believed early homo sapiens were unconscious. Mind functioned in an anthropomorphic state of undifferentiation from an animated cosmos, a process he called mythopoetic. He believed this mental state to be characteristic of the ancient Greece of the Homeric epics and of pre-Columbian culture, as well as the Old Testament Bible. He further postulated that mental states characteristic of religion, cultism, schizophrenia, and other extreme belief systems are leftovers or "vestiges" of the earlier unconscious bicameral state.

His hypothesis of mind did not gain the lasting respect it deserves because he conflated it with what have since been identified as incorrect beliefs about brain function and its evolution. We now know that all placental mammals have cerebral commissures; that humans born without them are still able to think, reflect, and self-regulate; and that cerebral functioning is based not on localized structures but on complex neural networks.

Nor is there evidence to support its basis, the hypothesis that ancient tribal and spiritual cultures were any less successful than more contemporary western culture, unless one defines success as the unique proliferation of population association with colonization and destruction of other cultures and the destruction of other species and the population. None of this diminishes the importance of the phenomenology he observed, however.

Freud and Jaynes divided these two states of mind into conscious and unconscious. Noam Chomsky makes a similar assumption when he claims that any speech or communication that is not recursive and is not expressive of reflective thought does not meet the criterion for language. It follows that Freud and Jaynes believed that infants and small children, whose speech reflects unawareness of having inner lives and of the psychological separateness of self and other, are not conscious. This is similar to the assertion of Chomsky and associates that infants do not possess language abilities because they use words and grammar differently than adults.

The conception of mind as a dual structure, comprising two qualitatively different mental activities, then, is not original. However, I have reformulated the mental processes in a way that is free of confusion and misconception about consciousness, dreaming, and childhood. Mental content cannot be observed directly but must be inferred from behavior, and in humans the behavior that offers deepest insight into the workings of mind is language, therefore much of the ensuing discussion about mind is about language.

Characteristics of reflective representational thought

The mental activity with which we in the western world are most familiar, which for the most part governs mature adult behavior and therefore is considered normal, is reflective representational thought. Reflective thought, what Noam Chomsky calls recursion when it is observed in language, involves both mental content and the capacity to contemplate it. It enables us to differentiate ourselves from others with some accuracy and appreciate their separateness rather than misperceive them either as aspects of ourselves of which we are not aware or as alien. It includes the capacity for symbolization, introspection, comparison and contrast, and the sense of a past (memory) and a future (fantasy or imagination). It enables the possibility of contradictory or conflicting thoughts; a kind of mental multitasking not available to persons shackled by belief systems and related reflexive behaviors. Reflective thought is responsible for the development of societies, cultures, and civilization based on implementation of the imagination and creativity of individual members, beyond stimulus-bound need satisfaction and social group adaptation. It enables us to tell stories that we recognize are fictions and not actual events.

Characteristics of primordial mental activity

Primordial mental activity, by contrast, is a holistic process that does not distinguish external reality from internal mind; the intrapsychic world of thought from an external world that it animates. It is a here and now process with no sense of time, past or future. It is concrete, not symbolic, a world of immediacy and enactment, not reflection and contemplation. The behavior it supports is not based on awareness of choices with separate consequences or conflicts to be resolved; rather, the experience is one of immersion in an ongoing action drama that moves from one surprising event to another. Dreaming is both the developmentally earliest example of primordial mentation and the one least contaminated by immediate reality considerations. It is interesting that for members of tribal cultures, dreaming and waking life are equivalently conscious and "real." Members of tribal cultures look upon their dreams as actual journeys of discovery, qualitatively similar to physical adventures or journeys in waking life, and do not make the distinction between waking and sleeping (unconscious) states that most of us in western cultures tend to do.

The concept of two equivalently "normal" and important mental processes on which we all depend runs counter to generally accepted beliefs that the earlier form of mentation is immature, non-functional, or inferior and unsophisticated, probably because it is most conspicuously associated with infancy and early childhood. An interesting functional comparison of the two processes that challenge this belief is that chimpanzees actually perform better on certain cognitive tasks than human children who have reached the age where they are capable of rudimentary reflective thought. The reflection and need to choose that characterize reflective thought may actually slow children down in performing some cognitive tasks, as their responses no longer have the quickness of reflex. This is the phenomenon Daniel Kahneman called fast thinking. Another way to look at it is that many complex adult functions that are beyond the capability of other animals, such as driving a car or performing sophisticated athletic feats, are learned from reflective thought, but once learned are taken over by the primordial mental process. The initial learning may be slow and laborious. Once learned, however, they become "thoughtless" habits and are done reflexively. We hear expressions like "the driver becomes one with the road." In such instances, "thinking too much" can be a problem as it can slow down or disrupt performance. Examples include some baseball players who start to "think too much" about basic activities like throwing and hitting that initially required sophisticated learning and practice but became reflexive. As a consequence of this regressive preoccupation, the careers of some star athletes have been ruined. Adults who relate to their children exclusively "by the book" in a logical non-playful way do not make the best parents.

Primordial mentation is not equivalent to delusional thinking

Some critics do not accept the fact that primordial mentation can be functionally adaptive, and personally and socially constructive, and hence is both normal and in its appropriate context uniquely functional. The noted anthropologist Richard Shweder is one. His doubts are articulated in a critique of Piaget's stage model. He confuses primordial mentation with functional incompetence; how the world is understood with one's ability to function adaptively in the moment. At the same time that infants' understanding of the world is shaped by primordial mentation, they respond accurately and adaptively to reality by reaching, grasping, bringing things to their mouths, struggling to stand, walk, and then reach perceived goals in terms of destinations in their immediate environment. This is impressive, limited by their level of motor development, not whether they perceive themselves as separate beings. This important distinction is elaborated in the next chapter, and depends on the undifferentiation, interdependence, or symbiosis between infant and caregiver that is normal in infancy. Among groups and tribes whose members are dependent and interdependent on such a primordial process it is not antagonistic to functionally realistic perception of and adaptation to the world.

Another way to gain perspective on the question of functionality and its relationship to mental process is to consider members of ancient cultures and of tribal cultures past and present. Chapters 3 and 11 describe how we in western culture tend to refer to the shared worldview of members of tribal and spiritual cultures as mythology. One would think that from such a perspective, if whole groups of people were blatantly unrealistic, or to be hyperbolic or delusional, the social system they embraced would be non-functional and would rapidly destruct. But this is hardly the case. We need look no farther than people with passionate religious beliefs in contemporary culture. As for tribal peoples, their beliefs or ways of understanding their relationship with the cosmos appear to have limited relationship to their functional abilities to navigate and survive adaptively and collaboratively in a natural environment. Their adaptive skills in their native environments actually surpass those of most members of contemporary cultures placed in similar situations, who may be logical, reflective, and adept in surviving in technologically sophisticated settings but are as clueless in natural environments lacking in such "civilized" appurtenances as "primitive" persons would be thrown into the midst of big city life.

It may be difficult for some to relate primordial mental activity in humans to the intelligence described in other primates in Chapter 2. However, language skills are not an essential part of primordial mentation. The next chapter describes the normal interaction of mothers and their infants that is called motherese by infant researchers; a complex choreography of eye contact and movement, facial expression, gestures, and at least in the beginning, very little use of language defined narrowly as words. The fundamental characteristic of these interactions is that they are a mutually choreographed, affectively driven, undifferentiated mutually adaptive mirroring that is not dependent on language as understood by mature adults.

It is important to remember that primordial mentation is not simply infantile, just as it is not delusional. It normally drives aspects of adult life as well. Parents of infants purposefully if reflexively revert to this process in the course of bonding and communicating with them. Artists in the throes of creative process are driven by affect; emotions they do not stop to name. They function in an "altered" enactive state we call the creative process that is undifferentiated from their work and is not logical. A similar mental process is often shared by lovers as well. Cults, rigid belief systems, and extreme religious states of ecstasy, all are driven by a similar process. The recent political upheaval between former President Trump and those who disagree with him and between liberal Democrats and the multitude of Republicans who loyally defend what from a logical realistic standpoint are false beliefs about reality and about others also illustrate a primordial mental process in action.

9

THE ORIGINS OF REFLECTIVE THOUGHT AND HUMAN INDIVIDUALITY DURING THE ATTACHMENT-SEPARATION PHASE OF DEVELOPMENT

The aspect of mind that makes humans unique insofar as we are capable of two distinctive mental processes unfolds as a consequence of complex learning during the lengthy attachment-separation phase that is unique to human development. It eventuates in a wide variety of adult human personality and behavior ranging from healthy maturation and creative social contributions in some instances to the unusual extent and virulence of destructiveness that is manifest individually and socially in others. Of most importance with regard to the process of intergenerational transmission, this wide spectrum of personality variation is reflected in parenting of subsequent generations of humans and the evolution of society and culture. It eventuates in civilized achievements, blatant destructiveness, and the much less obvious destructive behaviors that we tend to look upon as civilized achievements. These include the emphasis on the preservation and enhancement of individual lives that sometimes has destructive consequences socially, for other species and the environment, and in the case of unchecked population growth for the human species.

Our understanding of the psychological significance of the lengthy phases of attachment and separation unique to human beings and their consequences owes much to the classical 1969 three-volume work of John Bowlby. Bowlby wrote that attachment communication between mother and infant includes "facial expression, posture, and tone of voice" (1969, p. 120). Two years later, James and Joyce Robertson made a now classical film series demonstrating frame to frame synchronization of nuanced interactions between infants and their mothers and their disruption and reconnection during separation and reunion. Since then, assisted by the development of sophisticated neuroscience technology such as fMRI that measures interactions directly

DOI: 10.4324/9781003442318-9

at the neural level and can safely be applied to newborn infants, research into infant-mother attachment and the emergence of self and language has exploded. For an excellent overall summary of these developments, see the 2014 book by Ammaniti and Gallese.

The birth and infancy of mind

As described in the preceding chapter, Freud's groundbreaking effort to conceptualize the unique mental process of infancy and early childhood was based on his study of dreaming. The neurological substrate of this first process, reflected by rapid eye movements (REM) during sleep, develops in the last trimester of embryonic life. Its presence can be measured on the fetal electroencephalogram (EEG) (Schwab et al., 2009), Capellini et al., (2010) and is inferential evidence that, confirmed with adults studied in sleep labs, dreaming may be occurring.

REM sleep has been documented in terrestrial placental mammals and in birds as well as humans (Capellini et al., 2010), providing inferential evidence that primordial mental activity is not unique to humans. Anecdotal evidence from pet owners indicates that many people are convinced from observation that their dogs dream.

Prior to the third trimester of uterine life, the fetus responds reflexively to stimulation. The embryonic sensory-perceptual-motor apparatus is sufficiently developed by the third trimester of uterine life to activate the primordial mental system for intelligent assimilation and learning related to changes in touch, movement, light, and sound. The learned content can be measured in newborn infants (Partanen & Virtala, 2017). One of the most powerful catalytic forces consists of the musical prosody of mother's voice as she talks to her unborn child as well as to others, using language and other forms of vocalization. The manifestations of quickening or movement in the later stages of pregnancy that are unrelated to maternal volition provide mothers-to-be with inescapable evidence that they harbor a new life and motivate them to begin to interact with their fetuses with intentional and inadvertent vocalizations.

Darwin described the relationship between musicality, language, and attachment in 1871. Many others have written about it since: "The melodies of mother's speech are compelling auditory stimuli, which are particularly effective in eliciting emotion in pre-verbal infants" (Fernald, 1996, p. 71). At birth, the infant recognizes the uniqueness of mother's voice and prefers it to others (Kolata, 1984). In fact, newborn infants can distinguish mother's voice from a stranger's voice after hearing a single syllable in the first second of speech. Research has demonstrated that infants are born with preferences for things associated with the maternal voice that they learned prior to birth. Development of the language of primordial consciousness *in utero* includes not only the learning of prosody but also of actual words and sentences within the self-other undifferentiated system of consciousness that prevails at that time. Kolata (1984) demonstrated that infants who were read Doctor Seuss's *Cat in a Hat* twice a day beginning in the last six weeks of gestation sucked preferentially after birth when mother read that story in contrast to when she read a different Seuss story. Partanen et al. (2013) repeatedly exposed fetuses during the last trimester to particular combinations of nonsense syllables and discovered that subsequent to birth they recognized and preferentially responded to them in contrast to others. In the newborn, vision and kinesthesia join forces with these sensory modalities, along with the motor system, and these act in concert to create the mother-infant bond.

Although the maternal voice plays such an important role in human attachment via shared primordial mentation, it is not essential. Masataka (1996) studied a group of deaf mothers and their congenitally deaf infants and discovered unique qualities of motherese in sign language – slower tempo, exaggerated gesture, and more repetition – and demonstrated that the infants responded preferentially to a tape of their mothers signing material in motherese than when the same material was presented by other adults. I am not aware of any research on whether the fact that bonding in these deaf infants cannot begin until after birth has a particular effect on subsequent development.

First-time parents are often amazed, even shocked, to discover the seemingly reflexive facial expressions, high-pitched vocalizations, and unusual gestures with which they interact in a kind of mutually mirroring choreography with their infants, ways of being that are totally discrepant with how they interact with other adults. They are unwittingly reverting to primordial mentation themselves.

The newborn human infant is remarkably capable of imitation or mirroring what it sees. Trevarthen (1980, 2005) has demonstrated that only hours after birth, infants are capable of sophisticated imitation of gestures and expressions of adults who try to interact with them.

The behavior just described is colloquially called "baby talk" or "motherese" (Fernald & Kuhl, 1987; Durkin, Rutter & Tucker, 1982; Grieser & Kuhl, 1988) and reflects a primordial mental process qualitatively different from the reflective thought of adult life. This mother tongue is universal regardless of the particulars of specific languages, suggesting that its origins are biological, not learned. Ferguson (1964) documented its presence in six different language-speaking countries. However, accented prosody enables the fetus and then the infant to differentiate the native tongue from similar content in other languages (Werker & Tees, 1984). Mothers use language as though it were the infant speaking, mimicking its prosody and using the infant's name, or "we," and articulating what she imagines the infant to be thinking and feeling. The two speak together in a self-other undifferentiated affect-saturated action language.

Mother and infant initially function as a dual unity not only in these mirroring interactions, but behaviorally, as mother serves necessary functions the infant is unable to perform. The infant exists in a mental state Margaret Mahler called omnipotence, as it is unaware of dependency on a separate caregiver to perform the essential life-sustaining functions. The maternal functions are not differentiated from the actions and intentions of its own arms and legs. Infants will become upset and thrash about when a need or urge is experienced and mother is not immediately present to assuage it. As the psychoanalyst D.W. Winnicott remarked (1951) from a psychological perspective, "there is no such thing as a baby." Reciprocally, the infant is unaware that there is any such thing as a mother.

The learning that uniquely distinguishes humans commences well before the infant has the biological capability and the psychological security to begin to learn the language of reflective thought and the process of separation from mother that reflective thought necessitates and enables. Some of the learning prior to birth has already been noted. After birth, for example, the cries of Beng infants in West Africa are given meaning as expressions of the language of dead ancestors whose souls the babies are believed to embody. The mother's task is to decipher what the baby/ancestor wants her to do. The Beng belief might seem similar to some western cultural beliefs that the infant embodies characteristics of deceased family members (ancestors), but the western instances are more complex, as they combine the understanding of reflective thought with the belief of primordial mentation. Ashkenazi Jews, for example, imbue naming with a concrete sense of annihilation/reincarnation and believe one does not name a baby after a living ancestor, but most Jews would acknowledge that the baby is not, in fact, the ancestor.

The second mental process

The rapid postnatal maturation of brain subsequent to birth in other primates is in marked contrast to that in humans. The frontal lobes and myelination develop slowly in humans, over the course of the first two decades of life (Paus et al., 1999). During this time, the complex learning occurs that makes humans unique. Reflective thought gradually emerges from the matrix of mother-infant attachment. When the attachment phase is secure and predictable, the infant begins to learn that she has a mind of her own. When maternal attachment is secure, the infant feels confident to explore the world beyond mother and to begin to think for herself.

The "second language" that adaptively supersedes but does not replace primordial mental activity begins to emerge between 1 ½ and 3 years of age, and under normal conditions, the "baby talk" with mother gradually recedes into the social background (Johnson & Newport, 1989).

Self-reference in speech is a first step in development of reflective representational thought (Sharpless, 1985). The initial use of first-person pronouns does not signify the acquisition of self-referential thinking, however. First-person pronouns that appear in speech prior to about 19–22 months tend to be concrete and operational rather than truly representational. The infant initially refers to itself as an object using its name, undifferentiated from the way mother does. In other words, the first "I" involves awareness of the person as agent, performing action, and it is still a part of primordial mentation.

Until this time, the development of human infants and other primates is more or less similar. The mirror experiment devised by Gordon Gallup (1970, 1982), which was discussed in Chapter 2, demonstrated that many animals possess the ability to recognize themselves as agents as well.

At about 23–25 months, children begin to appreciate their separate being and the process of reflective representational consciousness commences. Use of the pronoun "I" begins to connote subjective awareness, and reciprocally, the use of second- and third-person pronouns develops as an indication of recognizing the separateness of others and of denoting social roles in conversation. The child begins to refer to his or her activities with a sense of possessiveness or ownership (my or mine) and to articulate associated inner affective states, marking the beginnings of emotional awareness. Whereas hitherto the child talked mostly about the environment, labeling objects and their qualities and describing activities, now she begins to comment on her own activities, reflecting on what she has done, demonstrating rudimentary representational memory and emotional awareness. The transition from the primordial conscious language of agency and doing in the world to the language of awareness of the differentiated self and other is manifest by the "show and tell" that is such an important aspect of early development. Labeling of one's body parts also begins around this time, also signifying a sense of body ownership, accompanied by mother-child body part naming and touching. At first, the name is not distinguished from the thing itself. Infants take great delight when they master the name, for example, of an animal. Calling something or someone a name is equivalent to controlling it or them, and most parents intuitively understand this and act instrumentally on their infant's behalf, fetching the named object if possible. Slogans like "sticks and stones will break my bones, but names will never hurt me" gradually reflect the process of learning that names are just thoughts. Most of us grow beyond exclusive use of primordial mentation and learn to respect others, recognize the difference between our wishes and reality, and come to express anger in emotional statements without throwing epithets or engaging in destructive actions. Some, as described in Chapter 14 and exemplified in Chapter 15, do not.

Stable use of personal pronouns and given name to distinguish reflective self from separate others, along with such developments as the ability to say "no" (and later "yes"), and to enter and leave the world of primordial mental make believe volitionally, is a gradual process. With this stability and security, the child can begin to function in a world in which the separateness of others on whom she depends is recognized, along with the possibility that they will frustrate her desires by doing things she does not like and the ability to sustain self-esteem and respect for the separateness of the other in such situations.

In normal development, at least in western culture, ages 5–7 appear to mark a developmental watershed. It is no longer possible to learn a second language with the prosody or accent of the mother tongue, suggesting that the learning that occurs is no longer based upon primordial mentation (Rivera-Gaxiola, Silvia-Pereyra, & Kuhl, 2005). In many cultures, it is around this age that the first concrete separation from the family and formal education commences, probably because the average child possesses sufficient reflective thought capacity to consciously strive to learn from the environment. Education changes from methods primarily related to fantasy, play, and group activities, all based on primordial mentation, and becomes focused on individual reflective learning. With the "three Rs," the child is required to distinguish the worlds of fantasy from consensual reality as articulated by teachers and codified in books, and to adaptively distinguish between the mental process appropriate to classroom learning and that appropriate to recess, where resumption of primordial mentation and fantasy play are encouraged. This marks the transition between a single mental activity, that of primordial mind, and the acquisition of an alternative that becomes increasingly a matter of adaptive choice. The individual, and by extension the species, is no longer stimulus bound!

As we shall see, especially in the discussion of destructiveness, this is not a transition all children are able to make, although the continued acquisition of formal language that is common to both mental processes may effectively masquerade this fact and enable some to acquire a false self. It is important to realize that even when the transition is made as part of a normal developmental trajectory, the capacity for and use of primordial conscious mentation and its language persists; it simply becomes regulated by self-awareness of what is and is not socially appropriate in a given context.

For a detailed description of this learning process from a somewhat different cognitive-emotional perspective, see the 2004 volume by Stanley Greenspan and Stuart Shanker entitled *The First Idea*.

10

THE BASIC PRINCIPLES GOVERNING THE SOCIAL ORGANIZATION OF SPECIES

The reflective representational thought characteristic of mature individual-centric mind, and the complex social organizations to which the acquisition of knowledge it has enabled has given rise, gradually altered the nature of human social organization over the course of human evolution. Each succeeding generation of human development involves a parallel process in which ontogeny, the maturation of the individual human mind, recapitulates phylogeny, the evolution of the species. The process is not simply one of recapitulation, however, but has involved social evolution through learning and the accretion of new knowledge by humankind. The capacity for reflective thought that enables humans to become separate selves has produced a typical form of social organization that seems to have evolved from the loose social organizations characteristic of primates, through an organization that is sociocentric and serves to sustain and equilibrate the group, to one that is primarily driven by the myriad of wants and needs of its individual members. The effects of the social structure now characteristic of humans have been both constructive and destructive. The actualization of individual potential is responsible for remarkable cultural achievements in the sciences, technology, the arts, and humanities. It has also produced a variety of personalities and parenting unknown among other species, including the problematic caregiving that "teaches" many of us as infants and children to become destructive humans and hostile, rejecting parents ourselves. What is much less apparent is that the emphasis on the preservation and enhancement of each individual life is responsible for an explosive increase in world population that endangers our survival as a species.

In order to place the evolution of human social organization in context, it is necessary to understand the principles that govern species social organization

DOI: 10.4324/9781003442318-10

and the contrast between human social organization and that of other species. From this foundation, it will be possible not only to understand what is so different about human social organization, but in a sophisticated way ask whether, however different human social organization may seem from that of other species, it still conforms to the biologically driven principles that seem to serve regulatory functions in other species. The question is fundamental to a larger evolutionary question, what biological factors, individual behaviors, and social organizations are necessary if species are to survive and flourish and what factors lead them to become extinct? Is all behavior that seems destructive to individual members also destructive for the species? And is all behavior that seems constructive for individual humans actually constructive for the species?

Contemporary theories of evolution – speciation and the life and death of species – continue to be heavily influenced by the work of Darwin 150 years later. Almost all theories of evolution are based on the assumption that it works according to a process of natural selection based upon epigenesis, the relationship of phenotypic adaptation to the resources and limitations of the environment and transmission of the most survival-adaptive genes or on autonomous accidental gene modifications and their effects. When adaptive homeostasis is disrupted beyond repair, in most instances because of external environmental changes, extinction ensues.

A good place to begin the discussion is the work of E. O. Wilson, whose 1975 book laid the foundation of the discipline known as sociobiology. As the name implies, sociobiology is based on the assumption that species' social organization is biologically determined. His early work is based on studies of non-human species, mostly insects. In it, he establishes basic principles of social organization including the critical species-sustaining role of what from the perspective of a human observer appears to be destructiveness. In his later years, he wrote about human society, but his work was speculative, not grounded in the kind of research that makes his earlier theories so impressive, and perhaps overly tinged with optimism. His early foundational work is discussed first.

Wilson believed that the societies he studied are sociocentric. That is, individual members of function not as individuals, but as subsidiary cogs comprising a unitary whole, like the parts of an engine, to coordinate to create and maintain adaptive homeostasis of the entire social organism. The members function to regulate the health and size of the entire population in relation to available resources, regardless of the consequences to their individual welfare. In this way, the species maintains population size and vitality within sustainable limits. Wilson's theory favors inheritance of the genes responsible for the most socially adaptive phenotypes, as this kind of social organization does not expend scarce resources on weak, diseased, unproductive, or aged members. Recently (2021), K. C. Burns, an ecologist, observed similar behavior in plants; a colony of staghorn ferns growing on a tree, each member of which appeared to be performing a specialized function related to maintaining the health of the entire community.

One thing that Wilson's theories make apparent is that sociocentric systems require, indeed depend on, what superficially appears to be the destructiveness of some of their individual members. In other words, purposeful destruction is an essential part of species preservation and regulation. It serves to regulate population in relation to readily available environmental resources and thereby to maintain species homeostasis. As we will see, part of the human difference is that destructiveness appears to have run amok and to be not only more pervasive and virulent, but most important, to serve no discernable species function.

In his first and paradigm-changing work, *Sociobiology: A New Synthesis* (1975), Wilson defined two types of genetically based population control mechanisms, based on aggression and destruction in the species he observed and studied. He called these R and K. These mechanisms function counterintuitively insofar as though they may be destructive to individuals, they serve to maintain homeostasis in the community in relation to available resources.

R behaviors are ones in which individual members of a group appear to sacrifice their lives for the greater good of the community. Their destruction serves a larger function of helping to expand the population. There are numerous examples of R behaviors in non-human species. For instance, ants allow themselves to be used as bridges to allow other ants to cross a body of water, and wasps lose their stingers and die in the course of protecting the hive. A 2019 experiment at the Max Planck Institute involved conditioning two African grey parrots to exchange metal washers through a hole in their cage for treats and then putting them side by side in separate enclosures between which there was an opening, but in which only one had an opening to the outside. They discovered that the parrot with the "cash" but no way to "spend" it would give it to the neighboring parrot so that parrot could get the treat. Sentinel Vervet monkeys loudly warn others of danger, diverting attention from the rest of the tribe and endangering their lives. Aphids and termites that are diseased or attacked explode, sometimes killing predators and in the process protecting others of their species. The male black widow spider sacrifices itself in the course of impregnating the female. Examples like that of the parrots might lead a human observer who conflates undifferentiation of self from other with empathy to conclude that such behavior is altruistic, but that assumes the capacity for reflective thought and differentiation of self from other which it is clear members of non-human species lack.

Wilson's other category of species' destructiveness, K, or kin selection, is characterized by acts of aggression and destruction toward others of one's species that tend to reduce the size of an overcrowded group and refine the quality of the surviving members. It is what is known colloquially as "survival of the fittest," and involves competition for scarce resources. The resources in question may be territorial including nesting, food and other limited supplies, the most desirable females, or tribal dominance. Dominance in males involves control of the most desirable female mates, and in females the hierarchy related to childbearing and child-rearing.

Before examining Wilson's later more speculative beliefs about human societies and their relationship to contemporary views of others that ignores or minimizes human destructiveness, it is important to take note of how easy it is to confuse human and other animal mental processes and fail to appreciate the difference related to the human acquisition of reflective thought and self-other differentiation. It is easy to conclude that the social organizations of humans and other animals are similar by misapplying reflective thoughtful human concepts to other animal behavior in a way that might appear to be empathic but is, in fact, anthropomorphic. Wilson used the term altruism in his description of R-type actions in non-human populations, conveying the implication that self-destructive behavior of individual members, for example, ants forming a bridge across water, originated from the thoughtful reflective consideration, let us say that might characterize a human who sacrifices organs to a loved one whose own are diseased, or more pointedly, the parent who pushes their infant out of the way of the bus and sacrifices their life in so doing.

There are analogous popular beliefs that some animal self-destructive behavior is suicidal, implying defining the term as it is used in reference to thoughtful choice, however misguided it may seem to others, to end their lives. An example of the misapplication of the term suicide is how the reference to mass behavior of Norwegian lemmings plunging off a cliff into the sea has become a metaphor for human suicidal behavior. However, the destructive behavior of groups of lemmings appears to be related to primordial mentation; absence of the ability to foresee consequences in their search for a new habitat when driven by the need for more space in which to expand their population. Some lemming communities migrate when population density becomes too great. They may try to cross a body of water without awareness of their physical limitations. Another example is group whale beaching. While the cause is not entirely clear, a current hypothesis is that changing environmental conditions force them to wander off a familiar course and into unfamiliar shallow waters. In other words, the capacity of the minds of these creatures to foresee the consequences of a survival-driven action may be limited. The nearest comparable phenomenon in other species to suicide in humans is when captive animals, especially in zoos, have been observed to bite or otherwise mutilate and sometimes even kill themselves, unaware of the larger consequences. The comparison to human suicide is inapt, however, as the cause is that these animals have been captured by humans, removed from their natural environments, and placed in ones that may satisfy human desires but have little bearing on the individual and social welfare of the animals treated as specimens. The nearest human analogy might be suicide when persons are confined in tiny prisons without any hope of release.

Cannibalism is another destructive activity whose meaning in human and other species is easily confused. The behavior – members of a species colony eating one another – occurs in all species and is not restricted to carnivores. Sexual cannibalism in which the male is devoured after copulation is common, as is intrauterine cannibalism. Under some environmental circumstances, members of some species eat their newborns. A thriving expanding colony of ants was discovered in an abandoned underground bunker that had been used by the Soviets to store nuclear weapons, even though there was no food there for them. They had fallen to the floor through a vent pipe in the ceiling that exited on the surface and had no way to escape. The puzzle about how the colony could survive was solved when it was discovered that they ate their compatriots when they, too, fell through the pipe. In non-human species, such behavior seems to serve positive purposes for the entire group, consistent with Wilson's concept of R. They may contribute to group survival and homeostasis under circumstances where provisions are scarce.

The behavior of members of the Donner party, snowbound in the Sierra Nevada mountains in 1846, is a similar instance of cannibalism in humans in the service of survival of the colony. When there was no other source of food, the survivors ate others who had already died of starvation. Intrauterine cannibalism is not uncommon in human pregnancies as well that produce multiple embryos, and would seem to be an example of K, reducing the population while enhancing individual quality.

On the other hand, there are numerous examples of tribes that, particular in the South Pacific, practice cannibalism as part of a cultural belief system that by literally eating the conquered enemy one can acquire his or her strength. These would seem to be a product of primordial mentation – the failure to differentiate self from other, not from species-motivated social regulation. Killing one's enemy and killing a diseased member who is consuming scarce resources might be seen as examples of K behavior, but not eating them.

Where human behavior becomes confusing is not so much whether it is governed by primordial biologically driven mentation or learning-acquired reflective thought, as whether it might conform to the biological regulatory principles Wilson called R and K even if it is thoughtfully motivated. For example, does human altruism – putting one's life in danger in order to protect someone else and voluntarily depriving oneself of scarce resources so others may have them – still serve the species function of R behavior that serves to expand the population even though it is thoughtful? This question is explored in subsequent chapters.

The human population appears to be expanding exponentially rather than remaining relatively constant in relation to available resources as seems the case with other species – insects, birds, and other animals. At the same time, in recent decades trends have been noted that serve to reduce population. Increasing numbers of women are practicing birth control and either choosing not to have children at all or limiting family size. And a handful of studies of controversial validity suggest that sperm counts among males in developed countries have been declining as well, without obvious external cause. Hikikomori is the name for a phenomenon in which young males in Japan are isolating themselves in their parents' homes rather than making families of their own and reproducing. Such phenomena satisfy the definition of K behavior that prunes the population, but are they? Requiring young men to go to war knowing that the probability is that they will die may serve a similar function. However, caution is necessary interpreting such observations, as correlation does not imply causation, especially in situations where the motivating forces remain for the most part matters of speculation, and unlike other species, humans are capable of reflective thought.

In the latter part of his career, Wilson turned from the detailed study of insects and other non-human species to reflection about human social organization. The result of his speculation lacks the hands-on observational rigor characteristic of his field work with insects. In *The Social Conquest of Earth* (2012), he introduced the idea that human society is governed by what he called eusocial behavior. His hypothesis was modeled after the organization of ants, a species he considered an example of social success because of their seeming ability not only to survive but to thrive under a remarkable variety of conditions. According to Wilson, a successful or eusocial species is one in which the members have transcended individual selfishness and self-aggrandizement and divide and share the task of population survival and growth among themselves so that not only the survival of a species, but its expansion is more important than that of any of its individual members. Wilson refers to eusocial species as "hive-minded super-cooperators." In order to meet the definition of eusocial or "truly social," animals must live in multi-generational communities, practice division of labor, and behave altruistically.

Wilson's eusocial hypothesis concluding with the belief that ants and humans are superior species does not take into account some significant species differences. One is the significant difference between the species related to organism size in relation to that of other species and to available resources. After all, ants are not the size of humans, and however successful they are as a species in terms of reproduction, in their relatively microscopic dimensions, they do not threaten to overrun the earth and endanger other species or their own species with extinction or threaten to exhaust or destroy the environment on which they depend. Wilson's definition of species success is breeding and proliferating. It does not take into account consequences for the planet as a whole or for other species of an infinitely expanding human population. Another is that ants are one of the very few species that have been observed to make group war among their own colonies and on other insect species such as termites. In fact, they are not an example of super-cooperators. Finally, and possibly of most importance, ants serve an essential sustaining function for planetary ecology, whereas homo sapiens does not seem to. Ants till and aerate the soil (without destroying its natural plant and animal life the way humans have), they help decompose waste material (whereas humans manufacture it in excess), and they transport seeds.

In the process of attempting to apply biological determinism to humans, Wilson also fails to note that the differences in maturation and dependency that separate humans from ants necessitate and enables the kinds and complexities of learning that no other species, ants included, are capable of. He ignores the effects of this learning on human behavior, specifically the evolution of human social organization based on the developing focus not on the group, but on individual self-actualization. Super-cooperators? We have become superindividualists; me-first cultures.

And what Wilson has not considered is that despite advances in civilization that enhance individual life, humans, both individually and socially, may be the most super-destroyers among species.

Richard Lewontin and Stephen Jay Gould have been two of the most vociferous critics of Wilson's attempt to extend his biological evolutionary theory of non-human social organization and evolution to humans. They emphasized the critical role of biology in determining human behavior (Gould, 1977).

The optimism that Wilson expresses in his eusocial hypothesis has roots in a long history of belief in the superiority of the human species. It seems to have originated in religious beliefs that we are God's chosen; a superior species made in "his" image. In its scientific iteration, it is rationalized with the belief that humans have evolved from our presumably savage tribal and primate ancestors to be a more caring, cooperative, communicative, moral, altruistic, and "eusocial" species. If human evolution brings with it associated problems, with our remarkable capacities humans will solve them and continuously improve our lot. Culture, science, medicine, and technology that have enabled us to conquer disease have prolonged the average lifespan to double what it was only a century ago and enhance control over the environment. These are the flagships of the conviction that we are destined for an ever-improving world and the associated idea that the human species will surmount all obstacles and flourish everlastingly. This is a contemporary example of the doctrine Herbert Spencer called Social Darwinism. But it does not take into account human destructiveness or the runaway growth of the human population.

The evolutionary anthropologists Richerson and Boyd (2006) and Robert Paul (2015) offer a new version of the old belief in human superiority and progressive evolution. Their interpretation is that the rapidly expanding human population is either a sign of progress, as Wilson understood the growth of ant colonies, or a problem for which, with our remarkable social capacities, humans will find a solution.

Recent books aimed at a popular audience echo similar sentiments. The title of Steven Pinker's book *Enlightenment Now* (2018) reflects his optimistic conviction about human wisdom. He views human nature through rose-colored glasses that seem blind to evidence of human destructiveness. Like Wilson, he believes that humans have gradually tamed our presumed once-savage primate ancestry and that as the result of stronger governments, education, cooperation among nations, increased prosperity, and increasing rights for women and minorities, war and violence are steadily declining and may eventually become obsolete so that presumably we will live happily and prosperously forever.

Yuval Noah Harari is another contemporary apostle of the doctrine of social Darwinism. He writes that advances in genetics and technology are leading inevitably to an ever more successful species, which will evolve in a humanoid or techno-human direction. This is what many people would like to believe.

It is interesting that in 2002, Wilson himself estimated that if current rates of human-caused destruction of the biosphere continue, half of all extant species will be extinct by the turn of the next century. This would certainly seem to distinguish us from ants and contradict his thesis that our species is uniquely equipped to survive. Many scientists believe we are in the midst of a sixth mass extinction, this one different from all the others insofar as its cause is not environmental factors external to species but is the rogue destructive behavior of the human species itself. This includes a combination of direct destruction of other species, destruction of the environments on which they depend, and expansion of the human population to a point that is environmentally unsustainable for life.

Once our thinking about extinction moves beyond the parlor conversation question of what happened to the dinosaurs, what comes to the minds of most of us are creatures like the dodo, a bird that primarily lived on the island of Mauritius and was last seen in 1662, and whose fate was popularized by Lewis Carroll in *Alice's Adventures in Wonderland*. Other common associations include the passenger pigeon, a bird that blanketed the skies of North America when the first European settlers arrived but was last seen in the Cincinnati Zoo in 1914. The final specimen of the great auk, a flightless bird that was easy for sailors to capture and eat for dinner, was consumed in 1844. In each instance, extinction appears to have been caused by some combination of human slaughter and destruction of the environments on which these species depended.

The rate of global species extinctions has been increasing exponentially. The Cambridge University Project on the subject has concluded that the "greatest threats to the human species are man-made," and the Future of Humanity Institute has reached a similar conclusion. Trisos et al. (2020) predict that climate change, a consequence of human activity, will bring about precipitous collapse in ecosystems and destruction of the wildlife dependent on them in the next century. The IUCN (International Union for the Conservation of Species) has made an impressive compendious study of extinction. According to the "red list" it has compiled of currently living species, the survival of 32 percent amphibians, 12 percent of bird species, 23 percent of mammals, 21 percent of fish, 57 percent of invertebrates, 70 percent of all plant life, and 21 percent of reptiles is seriously endangered. The bird population of North America has fallen by 29 percent since 1970. The 2019 *Global Assessment Report on Biodiversity and Ecosystem Services* by the Intergovernmental Science-Policy Platform on Biodiversity and Ecosystem Services concludes that the biomass of wild mammals has fallen by 82 percent and natural ecosystems have lost about half their area. In 2017, a statement by 15,364 scientists from 184 countries indicated that increasing levels of greenhouse gases from use of fossil fuels, human population growth, deforestation, and overuse of land for agricultural production, particularly by farming ruminant animals for meat consumption, are approaching dangerous levels. These alarming statistics are but the tip of the iceberg of what has already happened and what is predicted to come. This remarkable devastation of life and of planetary resources is the product both of an explosive increase in human population and of the very science and technology we look upon as the proudest accomplishments of civilization,

Human learning in the form of civilization, for example, science and technology, has led to hitherto unknown forms and magnitudes of destructiveness as well as amplifying ones already known. It has produced social divisions and conflicts between groups and societies primarily based on primordial mentation and more evolved ones based on reflective thought. It has led to social organization that is based on individual self-actualization and is therefore unstable with regard to the potential for growth and for destruction in contrast to the tribal organizations of our forebears, in which individual members were sustaining cogs or parts in the maintenance of a homeostatic structure. In sum, human social organization seems qualitatively different from that of other species. It is primarily a product of transmission and accumulation of learned knowledge, not simple biological evolution. Whether the difference is that humans represent an evolutionary flaw so that we are headed for extinction or whether, in ways not obvious, we still conform to basic homeostatic principles is discussed in the concluding chapters. Before examining the question of how human society and culture got this way, it might be enlightening to attempt, flawed though the effort might be, to reconstruct what human social organization might have been like at the dawn of the biological difference between homo sapiens and other species.

11

HUMAN SOCIAL ORGANIZATION IN THE BEGINNING

Inferences from remaining human tribes

It is generally agreed that homo sapiens evolved from primate ancestors. There were many gradual physical changes along the way, including developments in the brain, particularly frontal and prefrontal cortex and a center for speech, and developments in posture and gait, whose emergence seems to have been based originally on perpetuation of those changes most conducive to survival. However, the change brought about by neoteny, the lengthy postpartum period of immaturity and dependency, complicated matters so that the consequences of the other evolutionary changes are no longer so clearly related to species survival. The major step in evolution that comprise the human difference relates to learning and the intergenerational transmission and gradual accumulation of knowledge. The prolonged postpartum period of maturation that began to separate humans from other primates, and the dependency on caretakers and resultant opportunity and necessity for complex learning that results, seem to have been responsible for this unique human development. Associated with the acquisition of reflective thought, there was a gradual change in the structure of human society from the kinds of social groupings – herds, flocks, packs, pods, schools, colonies, and hives – characteristic of other species.

What were human beings and their social organization like in the beginning, at the time of the earliest departures from the social groupings characteristic of our primate ancestors? There remain many tribal cultures, some relatively uncontaminated by the insidious colonization that is characteristic of the expansive power of western culture, which lack the accoutrements of civilization and are organized around primordial mentation rather than reflective thought. As contemporary tribal cultures are comprised of members who have benefitted from evolutionary biology, it is not possible to

DOI: 10.4324/9781003442318-11

make direct or simple inferences from them about the social-cultural nature of early homo sapiens. Nonetheless, studying the language, communication, mental and social behavior of members of tribal cultures does reveal plausible evidence of an earlier form of human social organization prior to the kinds that can be documented from historical records that are based, at least to some degree, on the encoding of reflective thought. These tribal cultures provide a time travel window into what homo sapiens might have been like nearer to the "big bang," the dawn of our qualitative difference from other primates. The course of this social-cultural evolution is described in the next chapter.

Anthropologists such as Eliade (1964) and Nicholson (1987) have described the remarkable similarity among tribal spiritual-based cultures with regard to how they view person and cosmos. This similarity is especially impressive, considering that so many of them are small and separated, not only existentially in terms of geography and communication, but over the millennia as well. This is strong if inferential evidence that they share a common form of mental activity.

Cultures that are tribal or spiritual conform to the biological principles governing species' social organization and perpetuation that Wilson described. They can be characterized as sociocentric because their members function largely as component parts of a unitary social system rather than as individuals with personal agendas that may set them in conflict with one another in terms of goals and actions. That is not to say that sociocentric cultures are totally harmonious and without antagonism and destruction, but the destructiveness for the most part appears to play a part in maintaining the vitality and homeostasis of the community and its equilibration with the available environmental resources.

Consistent with the undifferentiated enactive structure of primordial mentation, the animistic mental process of tribal peoples may appear to westerners operating from a baseline of reflective logical thought to be unrealistic or mythological. However, caution is needed before jumping to the conclusion that their members are somehow less functional than we rational beings whose scientific minds enable us to appreciate reality as we understand it and from our limited perspective may even appear to be delusional. However, the beliefs of these peoples about themselves and the world appear to have limited relationship to their functional perceptual-cognitive abilities to navigate and survive in the natural environment they inhabit, abilities which actually surpass most members of contemporary cultures suddenly confronted with the need to survive in similar environments. We, in a contemporary western culture, are adept at surviving in technologically sophisticated settings that require reflective thought but are for the most part as clueless in natural environments lacking in such appurtenances. Understandably, "primitive" persons would be equally lost if suddenly left to survive in a big city.

Daniel Everett, whose work provided the data for much of this chapter, gives a remarkable example in his 2008 book about being awakened one morning by the members of the Piraha tribe, a highly skilled and functional social group with whom he and his family were living. The tribe was assembled on the banks of the Maci River in the Amazon basin. They were talking and gesturing excitedly about their God, who was apparently on the opposite bank. Subsequent to this shared experience, the members went about their daily routines hunting, fishing, and doing the tasks of everyday life. While such cultures, "lacking" in logical thought and some of its products such as science and technology, do not seem to expand limitlessly as do contemporary western cultures that tend to colonize others, they tend to maintain a state of homeostasis and equilibrium with the environment and its available resources. The functional difference between self-centric western and sociocentric tribal cultures is not between reality and mythology, function and dysfunction, but between relative preferences for reflective logical thought and for primordial mental activity and their respective consequences. This chapter illustrates the primordial mental process that members of the Piraha tribe use to understand themselves and the world they seem to navigate quite successfully.

These sociocentric or collective cultures do not differentiate a psychological self, separate from the cosmos. As a result, what we would call the natural world is animated and understood as quasi-human. It is not that members are incapable of making distinctions, but that the distinctions have to do with such things as individual differences, the ancestral world, and the day-to-day world; the soul or spirit and the body; and the distinction between the geographical and spiritual worlds. Ancestors are every bit as alive as existing members of one's family. Dreaming is just as real and reasonable as any other "reality" and is conceived as a particular kind of journey, involving time or space travel of the soul or spirit to another place or supernatural dimension or even to a self that has been changed, for example, into another person or animal. Such experiences are looked upon as ominous or portentous encounters that provide information about being in the world, whereas in self-centric western culture they would be viewed as informative about aspects of our separate internally perceived minds. The soul or spirit is not believed to be a psychic quality, but rather an essence that can travel in time and space. What westerners call death or termination of individual life is in spiritual cultures the permanent severance of the relationship between the soul and body. Similar though attenuated aspects of such beliefs can be found among Evangelical or born-again Christian religious groups in western society. Memory is lacking. Life is rooted in the immediate present, without a sense of past or future.

Thanks to the work of Daniel Everett, a missionary who turned cultural anthropologist focusing on linguistics (2005, 2008), we have a detailed account of the tribal and individual lives of the Brazilian tribe known as

Piraha. As was true for the original tribal cultures of our primate ancestors, the Piraha are hunter-gatherers. The tribal population is stable, consisting of perhaps 350 inhabitants living in a series of small villages on the Maci River, a tributary of the Amazon. Though small in number, the culture and language are remarkably resistant to outside influence, which has primarily intruded in the forms of Portuguese westernization and Christian missionary endeavors such as Everett's original initiative. Everett lived among them intermittently for several decades, first as a missionary and then as his orientation changed from religious colonization to scientific curiosity and study, he became an anthropologically oriented linguist. He and his former wife, who divorced as their orientation toward being there diverged, may be the only outsiders to have mastered their difficult language, which has a prosodic bird-like singing and whistling quality with extraordinary subtle nuances. His descriptions are remarkable illustrations of a social collective based on primordial mental activity and its linguistic reflection.

It might be helpful to review a few of the salient characteristics of primordial mentation before launching into a description of Piraha language, culture, and behavior. It does not differentiate person from what in reflective thought is considered external reality. It is enactive and dramatic; experienced as an immediate happening and not an aspect of mind subject to reflection and change over time; therefore, it qualifies as belief or conviction. In waking life, therefore, it is manifest in behavior, and the language it employs is concrete, not symbolic, whereas when asleep and action is blocked it takes the form of a dream. It consists of images linked by somatic-affective states rather than by emotions, which are not represented.

According to Everett's description, "Piraha culture constrains communication to non-abstract subjects which fall within the immediate experience of interlocutors" (2005, p. 621). He calls this the *immediacy of experience principle* (2008), and I would say it is a reflection of enactment rather than reflective thought. The Piraha live entirely in the present moment, in which reality is synonymous with immediate sensory-perceptual-motor experience. They make frequent use of a particular adjective/adverb to express something entering or leaving immediate perception, and if something or someone is out of sight, it or they are absent from discourse until again concretely present. Piraha language expresses what is and not what was or will be or what might be; there is no concept of time, past or future. It is what it is and is not used symbolically to represent other things.

Piraha have no trouble navigating through life; places are identified not by a symbolic mental map but by undifferentiated references to things like the personal activity that is or was done there, or by a concrete identifying geographical feature or a kind of vegetation or wildlife found there.

In this world of concrete immediacy there is no conception of passage of time, of time past, present, and imagined future, and no apparent sense of logical sequence, causality, or consequences. It follows that there is no memory in the sense of something that happened at another time and no collective history. This is not equivalent to saying there is no sense of things past, for there are accounts of what has actually been experienced by someone, but it is talked about as though it is a happening in the present moment. There is no anticipation or planning. For example, they do not stockpile goods for a future time when they might be needed.

This literal quality, lacking symbolism or analogy, was illustrated when the natives asked Everett why a visitor was spraying bug repellent on himself and he responded with a kind of charade by imitating the flight, sound, and sting of the insects, and concluded by slapping an imaginary mosquito, only to see the native observers turn to Everett in puzzlement and ask why the man was hitting himself.

It is not surprising, then, that the Piraha have no written language, which requires a degree of mental representation and symbolic capacity to construct, even if the words themselves can subsequently be used concretely, at times, as things, like expletives. And their spoken language lacks abstract qualitative descriptors. For example, while the natives are sensitive and responsive to color cues, they do not have abstract words for colors. Instead, they substitute likeness or identity. The object is not "red," it is called blood. They do not remember the name of a visitor; instead, he or she is dubbed by the name of a Piraha whose features bear some resemblance. Their language has few pronouns; instead, they refer to concrete and specific names.

Piraha language also lacks numbers and sequential counting or quantifying concepts, another instance of absence of logic and abstraction. Even after Everett and his family conducted months of classes with the natives, none were able to count to ten or add 1 + 1. This was not for lack of motivation, for it had been demonstrated to them that such learning might have value in helping them to negotiate more effectively with Portuguese traders with whom they have considerable commerce.

What westerners might think about as ideas, to the Piraha are things, placed adjacent to one another, sequenced by contiguity or affect state rather than by temporal or causal logic. There are no subordinate clauses in Piraha speech, no recursive combining of one idea within another in a sentence.

Piraha language contains few kinship terms, and kinship bonds such as marriage are loosely maintained and very much of the moment. This does not mean they do not care about one another. The most likely explanation is that they do not have a sense of temporal continuity or enduring representations of the relevant ideational commitments and their emotional basis. Someone who is gone from immediate sight or hearing is no longer a subject of internal connection, although he or she is readily recognized on return. While the Piraha show affect and are generally a playful people who help one another out in practical matters, they do not seem to be aware of feelings about one another in the sense of enduring representations or emotional states that are necessary for more abstract notions of attachment. Where feelings of anger might be expectable, there is instead action or enactment, usually in the form of distance or disengagement, and preoccupation with other aspects of immediate experience than the relationship.

Out of sight is out of mind. Everett's visits to the Piraha have been by float plane, landing on the Maci River. The Piraha are excited by this phenomenon each time it occurs and respond by making airplane models out of balsa wood. Each event is stimulus-bound and short-lived. It soon ceases and the natives lose interest in the models and the model making; apparently, there is no abstract or memorial significance, and nothing remains to be thought about.

Everett recounts vivid experiences about how Piraha deal with death and child rearing that are also consistent with a hypothesis of primordial mental activity including the absence of emotional representation, of a sense of time past and future, and of consequences. A woman died a protracted death in breech childbirth, while observers seemed unaware of the consequences of what was happening and apparently viewed her pain discontinuously as a thing of the moment and experienced no guilt or concern about her fate. Everett recorded subsequent dialogue with her husband who repeated over and over words like "she is not here now" accompanied by tone and behavior that conveyed his obvious distress but was devoid of awareness of the permanence of the loss or the need to grieve that would follow from such awareness.

Infants and small children are given what to western eyes is an unusual degree of "freedom" to do whatever they want. A westerner might interpret this as enlightened non-helicopter parenting, but it is reflective of "out of sight is out of mind," and lack of predictive awareness of possible future consequences. Everett notes the absence of punishment for forbidden behavior or protection from harm, both of which involve a sense of time and ability to think logically about consequences. He observed a scene where an infant played with a sharp knife, risking self-mutilation, in the presence of seemingly unconcerned adults. Infants are nursed until the arrival of another child, often around four years, and then weaned abruptly and entirely, often screaming for nights on end while parents, nursing the new baby, seem oblivious. Ordinary western conclusions about such behaviors that, for example, the Piraha don't care about one another are belied by their close community and affectionate and helping attitudes toward one another. Everett's interpretation is that they have a high degree of respect for one another's individuality and autonomy. He points to the degree of self-sufficiency adults manifest. This seems to me an implausible hypothesis, as they seem unaware of others' separateness and its consequences. It seems more likely that they lack an abstract conception of causality and consequence and are concrete and stimulus-bound.

It may seem contradictory to what I have written about the absence of mythology to suggest that Piraha is a spiritual culture, but spirituality need not be identical to symbolic awareness of stories and myths. There is no fantasy and no shared cultural fiction or mythology. Piraha mental activity seems devoid of the qualities of abstraction and symbolization that westerners assume when defining something as a myth. They do not make art or tell stories that involve imagination or fantasy. They do tell stories of a kind, but these involve recounting experiences within the sensory-perceptual lifetime of the person, but these are told as though they are happening currently. And yet Piraha believe themselves to be shape-changers, undifferentiated from spirits in the cosmos. There is an active spirit or dream world that they "see," believe, and participate in waking and sleeping that to them is quite real. Their attitude toward dreams is that they are another kind of immediate real experience or journey. Behavior that to the western observer seems to involve supernatural mythological beliefs and practices requiring symbolic capacity is concrete to the Piraha. The spirit world is experienced in dreaming and is contacted through transit into dreaming and through death. As noted previously, in the prologue to his book, Everett recounts having himself and his family awakened by the excited cries of the villagers gathered on the riverbank pointing to and commenting about an evil spirit called Xigagai, who they could see clearly on the opposite bank and describe in detail and was not a spirit presence.

The Piraha sleeping pattern might be related to the absence of boundary between primordial mental activity in dreaming and in waking life. They have no clear demarcation between a time to sleep and a time to be awake, and generally sleep for an hour or two at a time throughout a 24-hour period. This might suggest an absence of psychological boundaries between the two states.

As one might expect in a sociocentric community whose members are bound together by a mental activity that does not distinguish themselves one from the other and is basically biologically driven, there is a very close physical and emotional sharing bond between parents and infants. As adults, they are a tightly bound social community of individuals who share similar experiences and similar basic affect states, and considerable functional competence in the form of what might be called habits rather than thought-out procedures.

The Piraha have been unable or unwilling to learn other languages, even though they have been exposed to outsiders for several centuries, especially Portuguese. They refer to themselves concretely as "straight heads" in contrast to those who speak other languages who are "crooked heads." Their behavior and mentation cannot be a matter of genetic inbreeding of neurological defect, for although the Piraha do not allow marriage outside the tribe, it is accepted that their women are sexually active with outsiders, particularly the Portuguese traders. Hence their gene pool is always expanding and not entirely inbred.

As he wrote *Don't Sleep There Are Snakes* from the perspective of a cultural anthropologist challenging Noam Chomsky's theory of biologically determined universal grammar, Daniel Everett did not pay particular attention to the nature and role of destructiveness among the Piraha. There are some striking examples in his book, for instance, of the woman dying in childbirth in front of her husband and others who from a western perspective appear indifferent, and the infant who is playing with a sharp knife in the presence of adults who also seem indifferent. It would seem that natural processes, without active thoughtful efforts to alter them, mostly govern life and death in this small culture whose population seems to remain stable over time.

12

EVOLUTION OF THE HUMAN SOCIAL DIFFERENCE THROUGH THE ACQUISITION AND INTERGENERATIONAL TRANSMISSION OF KNOWLEDGE

The human difference originated from a combination of biological evolution – the phenomenon of neoteny and the acquisition of a larger more complex brain and a more complex vocal apparatus – and the evolution of a second mental process and the acquisition, accumulation, and intergenerational transmission of knowledge it enabled. Human social organization evolved as well, from one based on primordial mental activity to the multiple complex organizations that remain based on collaboration of individuals who function according to a primordial process, to ones that are based predominantly on reflective representational thought, centered around the welfare and needs of the individual rather than around maintenance of the group. As growing mental complexity enabled humans to leave records, steps in this evolution have become documents that our reflective minds can process as human history.

In the prelinguistic era, humans probably made sounds that became antecedents of words, at the same time they inscribed the images that comprise cave art. These lack a cohesive sequential grammatical structure. They are products of the first mental structure, and their communicative meaning is biologically programmed. However, from the beginning of speciation, homo sapiens possessed speech centers that enabled transmission of increasingly nuanced meanings from one member to another that eventually evolved into words and sentences. In the course of evolution of civilization, humans moved from a kind of communication that must have been based on spoken instrumental signals related to concrete events of the moment to simple signing. From the use of signs, the capacity to reflect, symbolize, record, track the passage of time, and communicate with others must have evolved. This enabled communication when the parties were no longer in visual

DOI: 10.4324/9781003442318-12

proximity but at a distance. It was part of a complexity that gradually included things like reflection and symbolization, phonetic linkages that unite speaking and writing, and the cursive writing that made the written word almost as easy to use for communication as the spoken. Invention of alphabets, consisting of characters that have symbolic and phonetic linkage, was one of the major later developments and made it possible for humans to construct sentences and written language. In the process what hitherto were oral narrative traditions related to the concrete undifferentiated beliefs about person and cosmos became the stories. Then it became possible to represent and reflect on what was hitherto belief or mythology, to recognize the difference between stories and real happenings, and to deliberately create fiction.

How did these civilizations and the minds that created them evolve from the stable mostly biologically determined social organizations based on the primordial mental structure of earliest homo sapiens? Cave art, the first enduring manifestation of uniquely human intelligence, was most likely the result of efforts to reproduce mental images. The oldest discovered cave art – the most ancient known homo sapiens document – dates back not quite 50,000 years, meaning that the remarkable difference between humans and other species has evolved in a comparatively brief span of time in relation to the history of earth and even the history of living species. The usual subject of this art is large animals, seemingly reflective of mental images related to the chase – the hunter-gatherer culture of the artists. It resembles the transient carvings of float planes described in an earlier chapter that Piraha natives made after each arrival of outsiders. A spelunker on a remote Indonesian island discovered a notable exception when he lived out what might have been a scene from an Indiana Jones movie. He spied a hole in the ceiling of a cave and clambered up to it only to discover a large hall containing what is at this writing the world's oldest example of cave art, dating back at least 43,900 years, about 20,000 years prior to the famous depictions of animals and humans in caves in Lascaux, France. In contrast to the realism of the French paintings, those in the Indonesian cave depict eight figures that are part human and part animal or monster, hunting wild pigs and dwarf buffaloes (anoas). Perhaps this reflects the beginnings of recorded mythology in the form of animistic conceptions of the world.

Nearly 40,000 years elapsed after the creation of these images before the date of the first traces that have been discovered of civilization. Evidence of Sumerian culture has been found dating to 5500 BC to 4500 BC in Mesopotamia, at the junction of the Tigris and Euphrates rivers. This is the area now known as Iraq. Evidence of civilization dating to approximately the same time has been found in the Indus River Valley in what is now Pakistan and Afghanistan, and the upper and lower Nile that became ancient Egypt.

Perhaps a millennium later, still prior to the advent of the Christian calendar, civilizations arose in the Andes (3200), and in the area around the Aegean

(Cycladic, 3300) including the Minoan (2700) and Mycenaean (1600). Signs of civilization have been found in North Africa (Kerma 2500 and Kush 1070), around the Yellow River Valley in China (Xia, 2070; Shang, 1600); and then the Zhou and Han dynasties. The breathtaking conclusion from this data is that human culture and civilization emerged more or less simultaneously in many parts of the world, suggesting it was driven by the forces of biological evolution, in this instance, the knowledge accumulating as a result of neoteny and the dependent learning relationship between children and caregivers. The pace of civilized change in the relatively brief subsequent period of recorded history and communication is equally astonishing by contrast, as though one abandoned the horse and buggy and put the pedal to the floor of a modern sports car.

The advent of civilization evolved along with the human acquisition of a second mental process, reflective thought, and involved a critical shift in human social organization that set it apart from the social organization of other species and that of tribal human beings at the dawn of evolution from our primate ancestors. Hitherto, humans, like other animals, congregated in small local groups – herds, flocks, packs, bands, hives, colonies – there are many names for such groups depending on the species. Civilization enabled a qualitative advance in communication from that involving immediate local contact to contact at a distance, and social organization expanded to include complex interaction and evolution among and between groups.

Biological forces alone cannot have wrought such changes. Biological differences – in the brain, the speech apparatus, and maturation (neoteny) – are fundamental, but the subsequent developments are the consequences of the uniquely human capacity for learning and the acquisition and intergenerational transmission of knowledge that the lengthy period of extrauterine maturation has enabled and required.

The Shabaka stone, dated from the first Egyptian dynasty around 3100 BC, is perhaps the oldest relic of the beginning transition to reflective thought. A major source of data for the period from 2600 to 2100 BC is the Pyramid texts, which were discovered on walls and sarcophagi. The Maxims of Ptahhotep, dating from around 2300 BC, the Coffin texts written on coffins from around 2100, the Sinai inscriptions dating from 1800 to 1500 BC, and the Amarna letters, 382 cuneiform clay tablets that served as communications between rulers in Egypt and Anatolia, are other early well-known historical sources. In Sumerian culture in Mesopotamia, as well as in Egypt, the Sinai, Canaan and South Arabia, China, Anatolia, Ethiopia, and Mesoamerica, alphabet-like writing systems developed somewhere between the third and second millennia BC. The elements that comprise written language differ from one culture to another. For example, hieroglyphic, hieratic, and demotic are concepts that refer to the inscriptions of ancient Egypt and combine pictographs (representational pictures) and ideographs. Ideographs and logographs or logograms are character symbols without an associated phonetic quality. They represent words, for example, Chinese or Japanese characters or numerals. The first pure alphabets enabling linking single characters, creation of symbolic meaning, and single phonemes emerged in the first several hundred years of the second millennium BC in Egypt. The first evidence of hieratic, demotic cursive writing appears during that time, suggesting the integration and continuity characteristic of language, written or spoken.

The prelinguistic era probably consisted of vocal depictions of images, analogous to the inscriptions of cave art. These lack a cohesive sequential, grammatical structure. They resemble the rudimentary sign/sound/action language characteristic of chimpanzees, and if they have communicative meaning, it is biologically programmed. However, from the beginning of speciation, homo sapiens possessed speech centers that enabled transmission of increasingly nuanced meanings from one member to another. In the course of evolution of civilization, humans moved from a kind of communication that must have been based on spoken instrumental signals related to concrete events of the moment to simple signing. From the use of signs, the capacity to reflect, record, track the passage of time, and communicate with others must have evolved. This enabled communication when the parties were no longer in visual proximity but at a distance. It enabled complexity that gradually included things like reflection and symbolization, phonetic linkages that unite speaking and writing, and the cursive writing that made the written word almost as easy to use for communication as the spoken. Invention of alphabets, consisting of characters that have symbolic and phonetic linkage, was one of the major later developments and made it possible for humans to construct sentences, written language, and stories, and thereby codify what hitherto were oral narrative traditions related to belief and mythology. As a result, it eventually became possible to represent and reflect on what was hitherto belief or mythology to imagine and to create fiction. After thousands of years, humankind has reached the launch pad of contemporary technology, the age of digital and visual recording and communication, and the quantum leap and acceleration of civilized development these developments enable.

Returning to the origins of civilization, in Sumerian culture in Mesopotamia, as well as in Egypt, the Sinai, Canaan and South Arabia, China, Anatolia, Ethiopia, and Mesoamerica, alphabet-like writing systems developed somewhere between the third and second millennia BC. The first evidence of hieratic, demotic cursive writing appears during that time, suggesting the integration and continuity characteristic of language, written or spoken.

Wim Van Den Dungen (2019), a Dutch epistemologist and anthropologist whose intellectual roots include Freud, Piaget, and Julian Jaynes, has studied the evolution of Egyptian language from hieroglyphic signs to more complex language. His analysis led him to infer an initial mental process very similar to the description of primordial mental activity – concrete, undifferentiated, unintegrated and immediate, enactive and operational, and animistic. It is the language of recounted adventures that are not yet recognized to be myths or stories. The *Epic of Gilgamesh*, from around 2100 BC, is generally cited as the first evidence of cursive writing and of records that reflect mythology in addition to or instead of concrete practical reality. It is a story presumably written about a real ruler. In the story, he undertakes a heroic journey in the course of which he encounters gods and monsters.

Western civilization commenced as part of a gradual movement north from the cradle of civilization in the Middle East over the course of approximately 1,500 years. Around 700 BC, evidence of a Greek alphabet can be found. The Roman alphabet and Indo-European so-called Romance languages evolved soon thereafter.

The major source of Greek literature is the epic poetry of Homer that we think of from the perspective of reflective thought as mythic. Homer codified orally transmitted stories of adventures that had been conceived of by a primordial mental process prior to the advent of reflective thought and the separation of story from reality that it enabled.

In his introduction to the 1990 Fagles's translation of *Iliad*, Bernard Knox, one of the foremost scholars of Greek mythology and drama, informs us that there is no such thing as reading or writing in the epics. Such capabilities did not exist at the time of the adventures themselves. Bennet Simon (1978) and Bruno Snell (1982) have speculated about the minds of these preliterate peoples from analysis of the records left us by Homer and Sophocles. The fact that the characters had names and histories and engaged in actions can mislead contemporary western readers to believe they connote individual persons separate from the cosmos, possessors of reflective minds. But in these epics, there are no personal pronouns and most conspicuously, no first-person pronoun "I." And there are no terms for body, mind, self, or gender and no personal pronouns. Entities considered separate and distinct in reflective representational thought, including mind (psyche), body, specific emotions, contemplated thoughts, and actions, are not clearly differentiated. What in reflective thought will eventually be known as mind is conceived of as soul, an entity neither psyche nor soma. In lieu of a language for emotions, their precursors are expressed somatically by affectively tinged facial expressions, gestures, and actions. Motivational forces are conceived of as external events and causes. Punishment of the hero by the gods for misdeeds is an enactment of what in reflective thought might be a sense of guilt. The gods who cluster around each, and their actions, might each be said in western terms to represent an emotion (wrath, greed, envy, lust, retribution, and punishment), often in conflict as humans in reflective thought have internal conflicts (I want to do this, but I should do that). Mortal heroes are distinguished by the particular gods and goddesses who favor or undermine them, in modern terms, undifferentiated projections. Odysseus literally navigates between Scylla (lust, wish fulfillment) and Charybdis (destructive impulses), opposed by Poseidon but aided by Athena in his effort to keep on the straight and narrow pathway home, as it were. No wonder the contemporary western reader is left with the impression that the panoply of Greek deities seems very much like human beings. Language is concrete, as evinced by the magical power of curses, proclaimed by the gods, to transform reality.

The Oedipus tale is about the crossroads of life, but it is unlike, for example, Robert Frost's (1967) poems *The Road Not Taken and Stopping by Woods.*

Those are reflections about critical life choices. Frost's poems represent the choice in *Road* about career and in *Woods* between life and death. The author assumes the reader will interpret the poetry as allegory or metaphor. Sophocles's Oedipus makes literal choices in his adventure, discovering the consequences in action and unable to reflect about possibilities in advance. Metaphoric interpretation waited about 2,500 years until the advent of Freud, who retold the story as one of child development in which fantasies of fratricide and incest are resolved by awareness of the law of the father, thoughtful choice, repression, and control.

In western reflective thought, we think of these epics as mythology, because when we read them, we reflect on them as conscious products of imagination. However, the Greeks of that time were recounting actual adventures in the undifferentiated animated way they comprehended the cosmos. A current-day iteration of this distinction that most of us are familiar with can be found in Christian theological debates about whether Biblical stories are literal histories of God, Jesus, death and resurrection, and so forth, or are parables or metaphors meant to have symbolic emotional significance.

Although self-centric culture did not have a major impact on western mind and behavior until around the time of the industrial revolution, it makes its first recorded appearance in pre-Socratic period Athens of the fifth and sixth centuries BC. Anticipating Kant and Freud two and a half millennia later, Socrates separated psyche (mind or soul) from body (soma). His student Plato conceived of it as a tripartite structure, comprising logistikon (thought or reason), thymoeides, spirit or passion, affects including anger, and the basest animal or appetitive part, epithymetikon, which includes what we would call violent fantasies. The appetitive part is described as sensory-perceptual, somatic, sensual, concrete, unbounded, and responsible for dreaming, very much like Freud's primary process and the model of primordial mentation. Like that model and Freud's primary process, it was believed to be the mental operation of childhood as well.

In India, at approximately the same time, sixth century BC, Siddhartha, the Buddha, was also conceptualizing a primordial mental process with sociocentric ramifications in which selfhood or self-satisfaction is an illusion to be dissolved in the quest for selflessness or undifferentiation of person from universe.

In approximately the same 500-year period BC, in the area around Sumerian Babylon, ancient myths about journeys, gods, death, and rebirth similar to and perhaps derived from the *Epic of Gilgamesh* were being rewritten in the form of what later became the Old Testament of the Christian Bible.

Greek influence on language and mythology slowly wended its way north with the Etruscans to the Roman Empire and Latin language and then to the Romance languages of modern Europe.

Another leap ahead brings us to the era of modern religion. The Roman Empire collapsed around 500 AD, and during those years, the Biblical New Testament was written in Egypt, and perhaps soon thereafter, influenced by it, the Muslim Quran. The millennium known as the Dark Ages followed. It was a world understood in a way that did not distinguish reality from belief. Any signs of individuality, independence, and reflective empirical reasoning were defined as evil and dangerous, a kind of mental illness then thought of as identity theft by the Devil, as it threatened the Church's sociocentric control over its followers. Mind was not to be differentiated from the mythological beliefs about God. What we now call evolution was God's creation of man. Deviation was defined as heresy. In 397 Saint Augustine articulated a view of human mind and inner life that included the struggle between selfless sociocentric conformity defined as goodness and what we would now call individual freedom, but in the eyes of the Church was evil bestiality or original sin. The goal of religion was a selfless function of persons as cogs or parts in the social structure as the Church defined it, with constant vigilance to root out the evil of demonic possession, individuality, *Malleus Maleficarum*.

In that era, people lived their entire lives in the small communities into which they were born and within which they were looked upon as parts, not as individuals. There was no need for surnames identifying them as separate individuals. After the Norman Conquest in Britain in 1066, however, the population began to expand and the use of surnames for identification commenced. But the surnames had to do with categories and attachments to larger organizations of which the person was part, not to individual personality characteristics. They related to things like lineage in relation to the king, fiefdom, and in many instances, the work the person performed. The origin of many surnames (barber, carpenter, tailor, fisher, hunter, skinner, cook, mason, and more) that persist today came from the occupations of these people that were then deemed sufficient to refer to them.

Around the twelfth and thirteenth centuries, the intellectual awakening known as Scholasticism commenced in western Europe. Saint Thomas resurrected the idea of an individual self and the tripartite idea of soul, mind, and body. However, there was no major social change in the relationship between person and social group until the Renaissance that began in the fifteenth century and the Reformation that began about a century later, around 1500, when the traditional rigid procrustean bond in which persons were more or less interchangeable components in a social group began to loosen. Humans began to be looked upon as separate individuals with rights, freedoms, and goals distinct from those of more powerful group authority. The secular or self-centric mode of thinking, with science and rationality as its masthead, initiated the transition from holistic groups in which people are component parts to society governed by the needs and wants of individual members and the competition for dominance with belief and religion that has characterized subsequent centuries, as alternative ways of understanding the person and his or her relationship to the larger world.

The remarkable shift from primordial mentation to reflective thought that is at the core of separate individual selfhood produced what we think of as civilization, the large division thereof that we think of as science and technology on the one hand and philosophy and literature on the other; more recently, social sciences that combine both. Manifestations of primordial mentation did not cease, however. They continued to make themselves manifest in such things as religion and many other social groupings based on belief rather than reflection, "fact," and logic.

In order to understand the shift in the predominant mental process, it is instructive to compare two cultural giants of the Renaissance, Leonardo da Vinci, and Nicolaus Copernicus, who lived around the same time, mid-1400s to mid-1500s. Copernicus constructed perhaps the first theory built around reflection and the conception of a universe "out there" functioning according to principles different than one's subjective beliefs. While his discoveries are related to astronomy, his more fundamental innovation was conceptualizing relativity. His model of a universe decentered from human anthropomorphizing replaced the accepted Ptolemaic cosmology in which the actions of the heavenly bodies were not differentiated from immediate human sensory experience and beliefs based upon it. He conceived of a reality separate and independent from the subjectivity of the observer.

On the other hand, Leonardo da Vinci, who lived in the latter half of the fourteenth century and early into the 1500s, seems to have been between the two mental processes. Da Vinci is at once considered a great artist and one of the first scientists and technicians. Perhaps, if it makes any sense to make such comparisons, he was greater than Copernicus; some would say the greatest genius ever. Da Vinci was a sensitive detailed observer of the world around him who depicted in meticulous artistic detail the earth, the heavenly bodies, the human body, and machines. From his imagination, he designed remarkable machines, many of which appear to be forerunners of more modern inventions. However, he had a limited conception of a reality consisting of external forces and independent interactions that existed independent of his beliefs, so he did not understand the need to do experimental testing and verification of many of them. As a result, most of his creations, such as the notion of a screw propelled flying craft, were totally impractical. On the other hand, recent discoveries suggest he had an experimental understanding of gravity and had begun to devise mathematical equations about it that presage Newton.

Relativity and the need to create a model that differentiated the internal operations of the self from the forces, actions, and consequences of an external world gradually replaced the dominant Ptolemaic anthropomorphic paradigm of the universe. Scientists began to study, model, and reflect upon an external world differentiated from the self. Only half a century after da Vinci, the work of Galileo Galilei, who lived between the mid-1500s and mid-1600s, was based on meticulous experimental testing and verification rather than undifferentiated belief. It was securely ensconced in principles of relativity and concepts of external forces of gravity, speed and velocity, movement and balance, measurement of terrestrial and celestial direction and motion, and the like. Galileo was convicted in the Inquisition for teachings heretical to those of the Bible, especially related to the concept of a solar system centered around natural forces in the solar system rather than around God.

By the time of Isaac Newton and his discovery of the laws of motion and gravity, from the mid-seventeenth to the mid-eighteenth centuries, the discipline of science, based on reflective thought, had been thoroughly defined and mostly separated from the hitherto prevalent conception of an undifferentiated anthropomorphic universe whose causality was attributed to a deity and defined by rigid religious doctrine. However, as recently as 1857, Darwin's hypothesis of evolution of species based on meticulous observation came under attack from the creationists who continued to maintain that God made man in his image. And a substantial number of people continue to harbor that belief.

Science spawned technology. And it was technology that produced the industrial revolution that began in the mid-1700s and was responsible for population shifts, including immigration and the movement to cities. These developments permanently loosened the sociocentric stranglehold of the Church and marked the advent of self-centric western culture.

The leap in civilization enabled by reflective thought and individual centeredness was marked not only by the advent of science and technology, but by sea changes in literature and philosophy. Shakespeare's psychological dramas, written around 1600, vividly exemplify the growing preoccupation with the individual person and his or her "internal" psychology. Cassius might have been an historian of the shift from animism to intrapsychic reflection when he remarked "the fault, dear Brutus, lies not in our stars but in ourselves."

In 1619, Rene Descartes, then a young man, was distressed by three vivid dreams he had one night and puzzled about how he might determine whether he was awake or asleep. This incident was the inception of his philosophy. In 1637, he published the *Discourse on Method,* in which he proposed his revolutionary understanding of reflective thinking based on self-doubt and questioning of the veracity of purely sensory experience such as is characteristic of dreaming, or primordial mental activity. His emphasis on the central role of reflective thought is characterized by the phrase "Dubito, ergo cognito, ergo sum" ("I doubt, therefore I think, therefor I am"). Descartes's view of human complexity, a person who takes him or herself both as subject and object of reflection, and who is separate from others who are also separate beings with their own centers, represents one of those iconic paradigm shifts. He challenged the undifferentiated god-centric or solar-centric universe of primordial mental activity in a way that changed the direction of culture and society.

In his 1725 treatise *La Scienza Nuova,* Giambattista Vico introduced a spiral metaphor to illustrate his concepts of repetition and progress, both central to the notions of time, memory, and linear change that are fundamentals of reflective thought.

In 1734, Immanuel Kant coined the term "the enlightenment" to describe this revolution in the understanding of mind. Along with renaissance and age of reason, these terms have become captions for this period of history. In 1787 and 1798, more than a century before Freud, he postulated a tripartite model of individual mind consisting of reason, understanding, and sensibility, which resembles Freud's superego, ego, and id, respectively.

In this process of psychological evolution, culture and society gradually made a quantum leap from one based predominantly on primordial mental activity in which the person is subjugated to the welfare of the group or species to one in which the actualization and then the welfare of each individual became paramount. Much of what we think of as the progress of recent centuries has been a consequence of the concept of self-actualization and is still evolving as our social consciousness grows.

13

THE DEVELOPMENTAL ORIGINS OF INDIVIDUAL DESTRUCTIVENESS

The interaction of biology and learning

The work of people like Jane Goodall (1986) and E. O. Wilson (1975) has enlightened us that Freud was mistaken in his belief that pathological destructiveness is characteristic of all species. Chimps and ants are the only other species I am aware of that make organized war on their own kind, and the encounters are accidental as they do not seek out other colonies but encounter them by accident. The rare chimpanzee encounters usually involve groups of males fighting hand and tooth over territory both desire. While they apparently use simple weapons to kill prey for food, I know of no evidence that they use them against one another in the way Kubrick's movie *2001* depicted. When large colonies, hives, or tribes of other species come upon one another by accident, they may fight, but such an occurrence is fortuitous and not intentional, and as Wilson explains, not pathologically destructive.

The problems unique to human destructiveness originate during the lengthy learning process that is part of the phases of attachment and separation that distinguish us from other species. During these phases of development, reflective representational thought normally develops, and infants and children ordinarily acquire a sufficiently secure and separate sense of identity to undertake constructive lives independent of caregivers. This chapter explores the vicissitudes of the interpersonal process – primarily the mother-infant relationship – that for some children eventuate in maladaptive persistence of primordial mentation and destructive misunderstandings about the self and the world that motivates destructive behavior toward self and other. The next chapter describes the most blatant and severe of these destructive outcomes, the psychoses.

DOI: 10.4324/9781003442318-13

Our understanding of psychological growth and development owes much to Freud. However, his understanding was limited by his preoccupation with fathers and with what he believed was the central problem of psychological development, the Oedipal conflict, around three years of age. He believed resolution of this conflict is the central determinant of adult personality and involves accepting the authority of the father, whom he viewed as the representative of civilization, and repressing one's urges for "selfish" gratification that might be disruptive to the "naturally" authoritarian social order. He believed that failure to resolve the Oedipal complex led to major human psychopathology, psychoneurosis. While he understood in principle that events in earlier infancy were also important determinants of adult personality, they remained in a somewhat mysterious subsidiary area called "pre-Oedipal." For reasons about which we can only speculate, he failed to understand the central importance of mothers in development, hence the role of attachment to and separation in the maturational process.

Over the century or more of its evolution, various psychoanalysts, including Otto Rank, Sandor Ferenczi, Melanie Klein, Donald Winnicott, Ronald Fairbairn, John Bowlby, and Margaret Mahler, attempted to revise and expand psychoanalytic theory to account for the importance of earlier developments, but a century after Freud his views about the infant's relationship with father and the centrality of the Oedipus complex retain considerable power in mainstream psychoanalytic thinking.

This chapter describes some of the problems that arise in the earliest stages of attachment and separation that interfere with mature acquisition of reflective representational thought. As it focuses on maternal problems, it is important to clarify the difference between responsibility and blame, and explicitly repudiate the unfortunate tendency to criticize mothers when children have problems. Simple understanding of biology informs us that regardless of contemporary cultural "enlightenment" about gender role stereotypes, mothers are usually the most significant caregivers, and it is easy to overlook that in the majority of instances mothers are responsible for the best in adult human nature when writing about psychological problems and focus myopically on the role of mothers. In instances where maternal problems have interfered with infant growth, it is easy to overlook the fact that these mothers themselves were once infants and children who were not well cared for early in life. Another way to look at the problem of individual destructiveness is that it is one of intergenerational transmission, of repetitive causal sequences rather than individual blaming.

Unfortunately, some of the responsibility for the controversy over mother blaming can be placed at the feet of psychoanalysis, specifically of one psychoanalyst: Frieda Fromm-Reichmann, who is widely respected for her successful work with destructive schizophrenic patients. She is best known for the novel written by a former patient, Joanne Greenberg, under the pseudonym Hanna Green, *I Never Promised You a Rose Garden*. Fromm-Reichmann did not have children of her own. She was very invested in her ability to provide her young patients with what, in her opinion, others whom she deemed deficient, particularly mothers and therapists she believed inferior to herself, failed to give them. She believed that the cause of the illness is the "schizophrenogenic mother" (1948, p. 265), the concept that launched an era of mother blaming. But it was not just mothers toward whom she was moralistic and blaming. Comments in 1952 about therapists who cannot form relationships with schizophrenic persons are distinctly critical and patronizing. She describes the schizophrenic individual as one with very special insight into him or herself and without actually saying so, implies that the therapist who is mature, smart, and sensible enough to understand such a person is equally special. In contrast, if the relationship fails to develop, it must be because of deficiencies in the therapist. "Psychiatrists can take it for granted now that in principle a working doctor-patient relationship can be established with the schizophrenic patient. If and when this seems impossible it is due to the doctor's personal difficulties" (1952, p. 91), not to the severity of the patient's problems. She lists in detail all the "problems" most psychiatrists may have that render them unsuitable to the task and concludes "the psychiatrist should admit to himself that – in his present state of personality development – he is not equal to coping with schizophrenics, if there is a danger of his harming them with his own anxieties" (1952, p. 94). In other words, Fromm-Reichmann was apparently a very critical teacher and supervisor, and her ideas about schizophrenia are suffused with judgmentalism. Her own teacher, Harry Stack Sullivan, was said to be extremely caustic, at times to the point of sadism, according to Robert Gibson, a colleague (1989).

Fromm-Reichmann is hardly alone among analysts in confusing personal value judgments and moralizations with theories of early development, though she bears much of the responsibility for the particular problem in objectively assessing the role of mothers.

For the most part, psychoanalysts followed the lead of Freud in believing that mothers had relatively little impact until Melanie Klein came along, and her ideas captured the minds of enough followers to lead to the split from Freud during the so-called Controversial Discussions in the British Psychoanalytical Society during WWII. The impact of these "discussions" which read more like intellectual warfare cannot be overestimated as they led psychoanalysis to accept the legitimacy of basic theories of development other than his. However, they also fostered another unfortunate belief that infants are to blame for their severe pathology. Klein's theory is that infants are born with innate rage at the world, particularly their mothers. Her theory bears suspicious resemblance to the Christian doctrine of the original sin. It is of note in understanding her theory that her son committed suicide and her daughter, who became a prominent psychoanalyst in her own right, so vehemently repudiated her mother that she sided against her and with supporters of Freud in the controversial discussions over the legitimacy of her theories.

In the process of development, infants need to learn to identify and control painful emotions such as fear, rage, shame, guilt, and more, as well as more joyful ones, and to relinquish biologically reflexive tendencies to enact their somatic-affective-motoric precursors. In addition to learning self-awareness and self-regulation, they need to learn to identify and respect the separate identities and initiatives of others. Good enough mothering meets infantile needs in such a way as to minimize the element of pain and distress to what it can comfortably cope with in the process of growth; in short, to learn to master its own body and mind. The implicit aim of good mothering is to keep the infant from having to experience utter, timeless, terrifying helplessness during the gradual process of assumption of independence and responsibility. Margaret Mahler (1968) called this early mental state that good mothers enable their babies to experience infantile omnipotence, and Donald Winnicott (1951) remarked on the result in a different way, that there is no such thing as an infant. The mothering person serves as an undifferentiated extension of the infant's own volition and as a filter and control for the infant's experience. Intuiting and satisfying an infant's physical needs is the obvious practical part. In addition, mothers need to recognize the meaning of infantile affects and somatic expressions and label and respond to them with appropriate names and ideas in order to help the infant acquire the necessary thought, reflection, and action to do it himself or herself. In this way, the infant will begin to develop an accurate sense of self and the sense of security, predictability, trust, and mastery necessary to begin to reflect on and accept the idea he or she is a separate self, alone in a world of others who have separate lives, and often separate agendas, and therefore might be sources of hurt as well as sources of satisfaction.

This is a remarkable and difficult task for a mother. Mothers who function in a primordial mental state that has been distorted by dysphoric affects during their own disturbed attachment experience do not differentiate themselves and their own mental content accurately from what they believe about others, especially related to hostility and rejection, and may attribute to the fetus malevolent threatening qualities and affects they are not aware of having originated within themselves. Starting in utero, mothers who wittingly or not do not want children sing negative affect tones to their fetuses, songs of discomfort, anger, and rejection, much of it in privacy where no one else can hear. Fetal needs may be perceived as hostile attacks, draining mother's body. Subsequently, these attitudes are enacted as responses to infant expressions.

In 1949, Winnicott listed 18 reasons for a mother to hate her infant and the consequences for infants and children who have problems with aggression and destructiveness. Mary Ainsworth (1978, 1982), a student of John Bowlby, devised a way to study some of his propositions about healthy and pathological attachment and separation, exposing 12–18-month-old infants and their mothers to what she called the "strange situation" experiment. It consisted of a one-way screen observation of infants with and without their mothers and with a stranger in a variety of combinations. She classified infant attachment behavior into four affect-driven categories. Affects were defined as psychosomatic experiences like crying and thrashing that antedate the ability to articulate specific emotions and their ideational contexts such as "I'm angry... or frightened...or despairing...or panicked...because...." In other words, affects are experienced in lieu of reflective awareness of specific represented emotions and their related ideational content. Ainsworth's classifications are consistent with the hypothesis that infants function according to the characteristics of primordial consciousness mentation.

She observed four kinds of infant behavior: secure, ambivalent/resistant, anxious/avoidant, and disorganized/disoriented. Secure infants were able to go back and forth between relating to mother and exploring the environment, and in the stranger situation were able to do some exploration without showing undue distress.

Ambivalent/resistant infants were anxious and passive at home and preoccupied with mother and her whereabouts in the laboratory. Mothers of these infants were observed to be insensitive to their infant's needs and unpredictable in their responses but were not overtly rejecting.

Anxious/avoidant infants were intolerant of separations and tended to be anxious and act as though they were angry. Their mothers were rejecting of them. Although they could not separate from her, in mother's presence, the infants tended to ignore her and treat her as though she was not present.

Another category of infant behavior, disorganized/disoriented, was conceptualized by Ainsworth's student and collaborator Mary Main (1977, 2000). These infants were anxious, disorganized, and confused; their behavior was often disruptive. They seemed caught in oscillations between approach and avoidance. Their mothers were characterized by the observer as frightening and unpredictable and showed no signs of consistent attachment to their babies. Main comments on one peculiarity of the language of these infants seem relevant to primordial consciousness, namely the presence of contradictions in their speech.

Lyons-Ruth (2003) and the Boston Change Process Study Group (BCPSG, 2007) formulated their own model of disorganized attachment. They tested infants of caregivers who behaved in ways that were rejecting and attacking and distorted the meaning of infant initiatives by responding to them with dissonant or inappropriate affects. When exposed to new learning situations with others, infants of such mothers manifested the kind of maladaptive and self-destructive responses, for instance, confusion, mistrust, and hostility, that observers interpreted as paranoid and that might have been adaptive responses to the rejection, attack, and confusion consequent to their mothers' behavior. Nascent efforts on the part of such infants to represent and articulate emotions of fear and rage were ignored, rejected, or attacked by their mothers.

Infants who have not had a stable, secure, attentive attachment experience not only fail to develop an integrated internally consistent sense of themselves, but their subjective world also consists of the somatic-affective precursors of rage, fear, despair, and insecurity, experienced in primordial conscious mentation that does not distinguish what is going on in the world from what is going on within their own minds. Such reactions are dramatized in action, and to an observer might seem paranoid, delusional, hostile, and mistrustful.

The children of such disturbed mothers are unable to make the normal transition from primordial conscious mentation to the mentation of reflective representational thought that is necessary for separation from mother and that requires an inner sense of stability and security as well as an ability to recognize that others are separate people and selectively learn to trust those whose intentions are positive. Instead, they perceive others as figments of their own dangerous imaginations. Primordial conscious mentation persists in situations where it is not contextually appropriate because the sense of self and world has been so severely traumatized and distorted. Moreover, actual efforts to separate, for example, to start school and form relationships with friends and eventually with intimates, subjects the child to a state of awareness of helpless dependency in a world that is not experienced realistically, but is perceived as frightening and dangerous because it is animated with hostile qualities from the child's own undifferentiated unintegrated mind.

The state of separateness is literally unthinkable for such children. Remaining in the unseparated, undifferentiated mental state of primordial consciousness becomes an adaptive solution; a kind of false security that depends upon not knowing and having to struggle with intolerably painful emotions. The next chapters elaborate the life consequences of such early failures of attachment, separation, and self-differentiation.

14

INDIVIDUAL HUMAN DESTRUCTIVENESS

From failures of self-care to the spectrum of psychoses

The aspect of human difference attributable to destructiveness can be divided into self or individual destructiveness, social destructiveness, and species destructiveness. Freud wrote extensively about individual destructiveness he called neurosis, arising from unsatisfactory resolution of conflicts encountered in the later stages of childhood and young adulthood, and his work and the great body of psychoanalytic literature related to it, which will not be reprised in this chapter, are devoted to the more severe manifestations of individual destructiveness, the psychoses.

Individual destructiveness is often concealed from view. We are often shocked to learn from the media that some of the accomplished public figures we admire and respect have struggled and been defeated by hidden self-destructiveness. Closer to home, most of us know people – perhaps even friends and family members – who have, more or less, difficulty taking care of themselves, defined as ability to construct and lead reasonably satisfying, self-sufficient, independent lives, to develop and sustain intimate relationships, and to create families of their own. And even "intimate" family members often react with shock and disbelief when their presumed close relatives suddenly become suicidal, overtly psychotic, or destructive to others. Perhaps some of us have needed significant help with constructive self-care ourselves. Such problems reaching functional independence and a constructive place in the social group are relatively uncommon among members of other species, probably because infants of other species are relatively mature at birth, the parenting they need is mostly biologically determined, stereotypic, and adequate to rear them in the short interval between birth and functional independence without significant incident. One of the few instances of pathological destructiveness in other species is sometimes encountered

DOI: 10.4324/9781003442318-14

among animals held captive in unnatural environments such as zoos, who waste away or even engage in blatant self-harm for reasons that are not innate to their species.

Psychoanalysis was created to study individual human destructiveness. Neurotic suffering is destructive to the self and often to one's intimate relationships, psychotic pathology is responsible for much of the destructive behavior that is unique to human beings, and individual suffering is often concealed from public view. This chapter focuses on the destructiveness associated with psychosis, especially the harm to self that is often hidden from the awareness of others by what Winnicott called a false self.

Less severe instances of psychosis are often misunderstood because the term has come to be associated with bizarre delusional hallucinatory ranting and raving and the need for psychiatric hospitalization. For most people, the concept of psychosis is synonymous with schizophrenia, images of persons who commit acts of mass violence, and people who live on the streets and often die homeless. Such associations are not only strange, but they are also inextricably entangled with value judgments. The concept of psychosis has been associated with stigma and equated with evil, bestiality, criminality, defectiveness, and other subhuman conceptions, since social judgment of deviance became widespread in the Middle Ages in Great Britain, if not earlier. Psychosis is a commonplace, not an extraordinary aspect of the human condition, and in its more everyday form hardly so bizarre as it has been made to seem. It encompasses a spectrum of conditions that result from inappropriate persistence into adult life of the primordial mental activity I described in earlier chapters, in situations where it is adaptively necessary to have achieved a separate sense of self operating out of reflective representational thought. While some instances of psychosis are obvious because of the behaviors that reflect them, for example, suicide, serious substance addiction, conditions we label sociopathic or narcissistic, schizophrenia, cyclothymia including more rare manic-depressive disorders, and borderline personality, others are often hidden from public view. Many such persons are quite successful concealing their psychotic ideation from others and have led lives of remarkable achievement and social prominence based on a socially constructed façade known as a "false self," so that when tragedy strikes in one form or other, those of us who have formed an image of the person through the media or even casual acquaintance are often thrown into a state of disbelief. More about this later in the chapter.

The second misconception is that the spectrum of disturbances I refer to as psychotic are manifestations of a specific neurobiological abnormality or defect, probably genetically based and inherited. This mistaken belief is also associated with value judgment and stigmatization. As this chapter describes, these conditions, for the most part, are the result of profound disturbances in the attachment-separation phase of development.

The generally accepted medical model of psychosis is of an organic condition whose mental manifestations are a meaningless product of a kind of electrical storm in the brain due to a defect or deficiency. That is not the scientific fact it has been purported to be. Despite decades of research, no specific neurological correlate has been found for these conditions. The organic defect belief dates back hundreds of years to long before there was a medical profession. It was used to justify labels and associated "treatments" that to our modern ears sound dehumanizing and horrifying, including the belief that the person is subhuman or bestial, genetically defective, lacking morals and the capacity for reason, possessed by demons, criminal, and more. As medicine evolved into a profession with scientific pretensions, such labels have slowly been replaced by ones that appear to be more "scientific" and caring because they are supposedly related to brain disease but reflect the unsubstantiated belief that they are medical and not psychological conditions, products of a genetic abnormality.

A brief history of the evolution of the medicalization of psychosis that will illustrate what I mean can be divided into three eras. The first of these, which I call Pseudoscience I, spans the eighteenth and nineteenth centuries, including the beginnings of medicine as a profession and its treatment of the mentally disturbed, and its first efforts to differentiate itself from the theologically inspired efforts to exorcise the devil. Benjamin Rush, one of the signers of the Declaration of Independence, was one of the founders of the first medical school in the United States in the late 1700s. He became interested in the treatment of mental illness during his training in London, and after returning to the United States established the first mental ward within a hospital. For this, he is known as the father of American psychiatry and is generally looked upon as bringing enlightenment in the form of science. However, he perpetuated many of the dehumanizing views about mentally disturbed persons and their treatment he had learned from practices common in England in institutions like Bedlam (ironically, a contraction of Bethlehem!), which housed and treated the insane beginning around 1400. Rush considered himself a humanist, and while he did not use "treatments" common in England like flagellation and confinement in chains in a dungeon, he devised a number of treatments that we would now look upon as torture and physical punishment, designed to exorcise the person of the imagined diabolical, bestial, or criminal elements. These included spinning devices designed to induce fainting, which seem like precursors of ones used to simulate extreme gravity conditions for astronauts; dehydration, starvation, exsanguination, purging with Calomel (mercury chloride, formerly used as a purgative, now considered a fungicide and insecticide), blistering of skin with pitch or branding iron, near drowning, exposure to extremes of heat and cold, and more.

Jumping ahead more than 100 years, the second phase of the history of mental illness, Pseudoscience II, includes the first half of the twentieth century, until shortly after WWII. While for the most part it was no longer believed that the mentally ill had been physically entered and taken over by the devil, academic medical wisdom was that the seat of psychosis, then equated with insanity, defectiveness, and criminality, was in particular body parts that might be removed. Organs removed with pseudoscientific rationalization included clitoris, testicles and ovaries, teeth, and gall bladder and thyroid. Note that the Biblical equation of sexuality with original sin still persists. Other practices included inducing hyperthermia with malaria and refrigeration to induce hypothermia and lower temperature to near coma.

As the brain increasingly came to be viewed as the site of the illness, and since it is obviously impossible to remove that organ without removing the person, attention turned to genetics. The eugenics movement emerged, advocating sterilization of "defectives." Most states passed compulsory sterilization laws. In a 1927 judgment made by the Supreme Court (*Buck v. Bell*), the respected Justice Oliver Wendell Holmes wrote the Court's opinion entitled "Three generations of imbeciles are enough." He stated that a Virginia state law permitting compulsory sterilization of those labeled unfit "for the protection and health of the state" was constitutional. The movement to legalize sterilization came from respectable academic institutions like Harvard, as well. These practices reflected views that were not seriously questioned until their ultimate and extreme expression, the effort to eradicate Jews and Gypsies, by Nazi Germany. The eugenics movement more or less disappeared around WWII, perhaps because mass branding of Jews as non-Aryan defectives and railroading them to inhuman experimentation and death camps became inescapably repugnant to civilized people.

Other medical-therapeutic practices that mostly ended in the years subsequent to WWII included insulin coma designed to produce hypoglycemic shock, use of cold packs, and most notorious, prefrontal lobotomy. Walter Freeman, known colloquially as the king of lobotomy, performed about 3,500 of the procedures, refining his technique for mass production in later years so that he simply drove an icepick into the frontal lobe through the eye socket above the upper lid. His most famous patient was President John F. Kennedy's sister Rosemary, whom he lobotomized when she was 23 at the request of her father Joe. She had behavior problems and social retardation consequent to deliberate efforts by Mother Rose and a midwife to delay the labor process while awaiting a doctor. Rosemary was apparently a sweet girl who was eager to please others. The procedure not only failed to help but led to further major disability requiring lifelong institutional care. The use of electroconvulsive therapy (ECT) continues to this day and new brain altering procedures such as DBT (deep brain stimulation) are currently being developed in institutions like Harvard.

Moving to the present day, which I think of as Pseudoscience III, the currently accepted medical understanding and treatment continues to be that it is a physical disorder, now called schizophrenia. The medically prescribed treatment is now drugs, designed to ameliorate symptoms.

In the second volume of his *Études cliniques* (1860), Benedict Morel used the term *démence précoce* to describe the characteristics of a subset of young patients that he associated with dementia. In 1896, Emil Kraepelin (1919) ushered in the so-called modern era of scientific understanding when he published his famous text on dementia praecox, a progressive mental deterioration that he believed had its onset in late adolescence and early adulthood, which he believed to be an organic disease of the frontal lobes, despite, by his own admission, the absence of any detectable lesion. In 1911, Eugen Bleuler ushered in our current medical-scientific understanding when he renamed Kraepelin's dementia praecox "schizophrenia." Bleuler believed the primary symptoms were the consequence of hereditary neural degeneracy, and in his 1911 *Textbook of Psychiatry*, he recommended sterilization of schizophrenics to avoid propagating this organic taint:

> The more severely burdened should not propagate themselves… If we do nothing but make mental and physical cripples capable of propagating themselves, and the healthy stocks have to limit the number of their children because so much has to be done for the maintenance of others, if natural selection is generally suppressed, then unless we will get new measures our race must rapidly deteriorate.
>
> *(p. 214)*

World War II was a watershed in the treatment of psychosis. One of its sequelae was the emergence of three fields that gradually allied themselves with psychiatry: neuroscience, the pharmaceutical industry, and the health care insurance industry. These strange bedfellows soon discovered a common identity and financial interest and informally joined forces profiting immensely by literally selling to the public the belief that mental ills are physical ills that are treatable by chemical means. Research at Sandoz labs soon after the war led to the belief that a "model psychosis" could be induced and studied with LSD and the creation of Chlorpromazine, a drug that seemed capable of mitigating the symptoms of psychosis. The rapidly expanding pharmaceutical industry recognized that the creation of new drugs to treat the symptoms of psychiatric illness might be a hugely profitable enterprise. Psychiatrists realized that psychopharmacology, enabling rapid treatment of a large number of patients, could be a hugely profitable feel-good enterprise. And the insurance industry identified a new class of treatments from which it might profit.

The banner slogan of the new field of neuroscience was articulated by Sir Francis Crick, the codiscoverer of the structure of DNA, in the introduction to his 1994 book *The Astonishing Hypothesis*:

> The astonishing hypothesis is that you, your joys and your sorrows, your memories and your ambitions, your sense of identity and free will, are in fact nothing more than the behavior of a vast assembly of nerve cells and their associated molecules.

To rephrase Lewis Carroll's Alice, "You're nothing but a pack of neurons."

In 1952, a committee of the American Psychiatric Association wrote the bible of psychiatry, the *Diagnostic and Statistical Manual* (DSM), giving psychiatry its first legitimate medical manual. It consisted of naming and defining patterns of mind and behavior they believed abnormal as diseases regardless of the fact that almost none of them had an underlying medical-somatic cause. The manual has undergone five major and several minor revisions in the intervening three-quarters of the century, and while some of these diagnostic labels like schizophrenia, depression, and bipolar disorder have remained more or less constant, others come and go as fashions have changed. The most egregious example of the social judgments underlying DSM "science" is homosexuality. In the first 1952 edition, homosexuality was listed among the sociopathic disorders. Needless to say, in common parlance, sociopathy is more or less equated with criminality. It remained a DSM diagnosis until 1974 when it was "de-criminalized" and replaced with a less onerous disease label, not because of new scientific findings, but by a vote of the membership of the American Psychiatric Association, and relabeled "sexual orientation disturbance." This is but one instance of many DSM diagnoses that are instances of judgmental labeling of conditions as physical ills.

Chapter 2 of the now current DSM-5 describes schizophrenia as the result of a genetically determined neurological disorder that begins at predictable developmental stages, childhood or late adolescence and early adulthood. Contrary to the axiom of the psychiatric bible, however, and despite extensive and expensive research spanning many decades, funded by the quartet that stands most to profit from it, especially the pharmaceutical industry, it has not been proven that the DSM "disease" called schizophrenia has a specific identifiable physical substrate. There are no consistent findings in all or even most cases, and in individual cases none are of a magnitude that in controlled studies distinguish a schizophrenic person from a control population. Moreover, the findings that are cited in some instances might be related to impairment secondary to the drugs such patients are almost always given or to the mental and social dilapidation that characterizes chronic cases that have not had the benefit of significant psychosocial intervention.

It is the genetic findings that most proponents of the organic hypothesis cite as evidence. These are based on identical twin studies in instances of adoption. Joseph (2003) has made an exhaustive analysis of the original studies and concluded that there is no convincing evidence that genetic factors account for more than a small percentage of the variance among schizophrenics. And despite exhaustive genetic analyses, no specific causal gene or combination of genes have been found as is the case, for example, in Huntington's disease. Thomas Insel, former director of NIMH, whose tenure was dedicated to an expensive and exhaustive search for the genetic cause of schizophrenia, had this to say in his 2022 book: "Each of those [genetic] variants that have been discovered just account for a tiny, tiny amount of risk, so in aggregate, they're probably significant, but you have to put a hundred of them together," he said. "So, we started doing bigger and bigger studies to find smaller and smaller effects." The most plausible conclusion from genetic research is that it would take a remarkable combination of multiple factors to produce a single case, and the findings could account for but a few cases of psychosis. All we know after these decades of exhaustive expensive genetic research is that genetic factors of low-level individual potency appear to enhance risk in some instances but are not determinative. An alternative hypothesis that is not considered to account for those instances, in which there is an identifiable family history of illness, is that of intergenerational transmission of disturbance in the attachment-separation phase of development.

On April 2, 2013, Steven Hyman, former director of the National Institute of Mental Health, referred to DSM in a post on the website of the Dana Foundation for brain research as "an absolute scientific nightmare ... totally wrong." In an April 29, 2013, post on the National Institute of Health website, his successor, Thomas Insel, said: "Unlike our definitions of ischemic heart disease, lymphoma, or AIDS, the DSM diagnoses are based on a consensus about clusters of clinical symptoms, not any objective laboratory measure... symptoms alone rarely indicate the best choice of treatment." Allen Frances, chair of the task force that published the fourth edition of DSM, subsequently became disenchanted with its legitimacy. In 2014, he wrote that DSM diagnoses are nothing more than descriptive observations and judgments, not research-validated medical diseases.

The obvious hypothesis most remain curiously reluctant to consider seriously is that many, if not most, instances of schizophrenia are predominantly the consequences of early psychological developmental disturbances. They usually come to social attention at one of three nodal points in the life cycle, each of which can be characterized as a transition point in the maturational process of separation and individuation; in other words, the life transition milestones that most closely recapitulate the separation phase of infancy. The first is when children cannot separate sufficiently from their primary relationship and home to begin school. The second is when adolescents or young adults cannot successfully leave home to begin advanced education or work. Finally, there are adults who have formally left home and live on their own and appear to function more or less independently but are unable to form and sustain a close relationship and begin families of their own and/or to form a stable productive work life, or in the case of women, are faced with the stresses of pregnancy and childbirth that have got to stir associations to their own childhood experiences with mothers.

Failure of the first separation produces child psychosis. Failure of the second separation, leaving home for advanced education and/or a working career, produces overt signs and symptoms that we call schizophrenia as well as other behaviors we associate with severe mental ills. These include the perpetrators of school shooting tragedies; crimes that are mostly committed by young men in their late teens or early 20s who are about to graduate or have recently graduated high school. The predominant emotion underlying schizophrenia is rage, which is not surprising given the trauma such individuals have suffered during the early attachment-separation phase of life. Homicides, suicides, and drug addictions often occur at this time of life, as well.

Failure at the third stage of separation is typical of a destructive condition of which most people are much less aware; a psychotic personality organization that until that time had been mostly concealed from the social world of the sufferer by the superficial presentation of a false self. Such a façade is constructed based on the belief that if others knew who the person is "really", they would be hostile and rejecting. Such a belief is an understandable outgrowth of the actual experience the person had as an infant. The person retains sufficient sense of reality to intuit and conform to ordinary social expectations unless stressed by the demands of a close relationship. The British psychoanalyst Donald Winnicott coined the term "false self" in 1960, but it is a misnomer insofar as the construct is an integral part of the psychotic personality disorder and adaptive process. While this façade often employs many of the person's abilities, it is rooted in a wish to comply with imagined demands rather than in awareness of the person's true emotional needs and desires, and as it moves the person further and further away from his or her own fundamental needs, it contains the seeds of self-destruction and exposure.

The false self may be extremely effective. From an external vantage point, the person may seem unusually gifted and accomplished and even contribute significantly to society. It is only in intimate personal settings such as a close relationship or a psychoanalytic treatment situation that the psychosis becomes apparent. From time to time, we read of persons of public importance and significant accomplishment whose destructive private lives have hitherto been hidden from others. So, it comes as such a shock, for example, when a well-known successful person commits suicide, or is found to be a drug or alcohol addict, or otherwise requires mental hospitalization.

Depression or more overt psychosis following pregnancy is another example. It is not surprising that the mother-infant relationship is especially taxing for women who themselves have been traumatized at that early stage of life. If and when such people come to psychiatric attention because of suffering they experience or inflict on others, they are usually labeled with such names as borderline, schizoid, postpartum psychosis, sociopathic or narcissistic personality, and drug or alcohol addicted. In including addictions, I am not suggesting that all addictive behavior is a reflection of psychosis, as some are clearly socially determined by the misuse of addicting drugs that is endemic to our drug-dependent society. The false self-configuration is illustrated in the next chapter by three case reports.

In summary, individual self-destructive mentation and behavior, whether psychotic or in the form of more ordinary garden-variety failures, is usually the result of failures of the parent-infant relationship during the attachment-separation phase of development. The failures and deficiencies of parenting reflect and recapitulate the way parents themselves were treated as infants, so that they have become adults who are incapable of making consistent loving attachments to others, and the parents, once victims, visit upon their children their inappropriate anachronistic responses to the ways in which they themselves were parented. This cycle represents the intergenerational transmission of mental illness, a destructive cycle that repeats itself through human interaction and learning, not genetic transmission.

15

INDIVIDUAL HUMAN DESTRUCTIVENESS

Four patients and a former president

Individual destructiveness that is uniquely human and that is a consequence of severe disturbances in infantile and early childhood attachment and separation is much more common than is generally appreciated. This chapter recounts the stories of four former patients who had the benefit of intensive long-term psychoanalytic therapy for psychosis and concludes with a discussion of former President Donald Trump, using quotes from his speeches and tweets as well as first-hand descriptions from others.

None of the patients came to attention because of public acts of destruction. In fact, all of them were generally perceived as productive contributors to society, at least two exceptionally so. The purpose of the patient presentations is to illustrate that psychosis exists on a spectrum of severity and afflicts far more people than is generally appreciated. They are also intended to illustrate the false self that I described in the preceding chapter that effectively shields the self-destructive illness from public view, often even from the awareness of persons who are considered to be close friends and acquaintances. At least one of the patients would certainly have committed suicide had it not been for her therapy, and others expressed the belief they would have as well. One of the persons struggled throughout much of his life with the urge to murder persons close to him. These persons exemplify a large segment of the population that is invisible to most of us as they tend to live what might be called lives of quiet desperation, more or less successfully hidden from the public eye because of the success of their false selves. The account of President Trump is intended to call attention to someone who has enjoyed much social and personal success despite his destructiveness and therefore, as mental health and illness are social value judgment, and he has not sought or required such help, cannot be diagnosed as mentally ill. It will be introduced separately.

DOI: 10.4324/9781003442318-15

Before proceeding, a word about methodology. Can valid historical assumptions and conclusions about the external world be derived from the reports of persons who have difficulty distinguishing external from internal reality and who tend to hold others accountable for feelings and attitudes they are unable to perceive as originating within themselves? One of the major investigative tools a psychoanalyst uses is called transference analysis. History is to be found in repetition or reenactment at least as much as in direct oral narrative; the embeddedness of the past in actions in the present relationship between patient and analyst. As Santayana said, those who do not understand the past are doomed to repeat it. In the early undifferentiated unintegrated state of development characteristic of the attachment phase of development that I have described in preceding chapters, the psyche animates the external world with ideas, attitudes, feelings, and beliefs that are not yet recognized as being one's own, and conversely, with many beliefs and actions that have been learned and internalized from the problematic caregiver as coping mechanisms. The psychoanalyst learns in the course of a personal analysis to understand his or her mind well enough to comprehend when a patient is functioning in a self-other undifferentiated state and attributing disowned qualities of self to the analyst and when the patient's assessments of the analyst, though painful to hear, may be true. Examples of this kind of adaptation can be seen in the strange situation experiment described in Chapter 2 in which the infants of disturbed mothers are seen both as treating the stranger as though she were the mother and as acting like the mother herself. In psychoanalytic therapy, identification of these distortions of the relationship between patient and therapist enables gradual construction of a sense of what is actually transpiring between patient and analyst and gradual reconstruction – not usually veridical memory – of what the early attachment-separation relationship must have been like.

Dorothy

Dorothy was an unmarried professor in her late 30s, whose work in a social relations field was already internationally known, when she was referred to me in the throes of a severe regressive episode during which she had isolated herself in her apartment, did not bathe, eat, or take out trash, and engaged in physical self-mutilation. She had hoarded pills, and although she agreed to come to see me, she had thoroughly rationalized the wisdom of killing herself. As someone with experience working with suicidal individuals, I concluded after talking with her that it was more than likely she would do so. I felt my hands were tied because I knew if I told her she had to be hospitalized, she would refuse to see me, she had committed no social act sufficient to justify legal means to hospitalize her, and she had no close relatives in a position to take responsibility for her should I choose to appeal to them for help. As far as I could ascertain, and subsequent experience proved me correct, no one in her life had any idea of how disturbed she was. Outside her successful professional work, the few people she called friends sounded very disturbed themselves, and to the extent they knew anything about her thinking either believed similar things themselves or did not believe her actions were unusual. In fact, some years later, the closest of these "friends" committed suicide.

Dorothy was initially convinced I had a knife in my desk drawer and was about to kill her. I had to leave the office door open and tell her that she could leave at any time. Subsequently, for long periods of time, she was convinced that any spontaneous movements or expressions I made during our sessions were sexual-sadistic preludes to attacking her. Among her delusions was the belief that if she shot herself in the head, a beautiful flower garden would grow there. She harbored an even stranger belief that I only learned about well along in our work, that she literally had no body and no emotions. She could actually look in the mirror and not see anything except her head, and she had such science fiction-like belief as that she had two separate circulatory systems and that she was a disembodied head.

If you are expecting from this description to hear about a dilapidated bizarre person, you will be surprised to learn that in her daily life, Dorothy was an accomplished academic, a respected teacher, and internationally recognized authority on adolescent psychology. As we eventually discovered, consistent with her delusions, she did not believe that any of what she taught others applied to her, and worse, could not grasp the fact that she did not practice what she preached was a gross contradiction and a matter about which to be concerned. It had long ago become her *modus operandi*. She had no intimate relationships; for many years, none of her friends could understand why she was in therapy, and she made no effort to tell them, leading them to believe that I was exploiting her, an idea consistent with some of her own thinking.

Dorothy's childhood was extremely traumatic. Her mother so profoundly rejected her at birth that she refused to believe Dorothy was her baby, to remember her name, and threatened to give her away. Her mother and her aunt, who was another caregiver, often called her by someone else's name as she got older and reproached her if she objected. Mother treated Dorothy with a combination of neglect and abuse. When Dorothy sustained a compound fracture of her arm in which bone protruded through skin, mother was so upset she had to leave the room. It was many years before Dorothy realized the extent of mother's hostile rejecting behavior, as she internalized many of her mother's attacking attitudes which seemed to her normal and turned them on herself, for example, rejecting her body, her emotions, and her need for a human attachment and believing that her multiple forms of self-harm were good for her.

Dorothy was an exceptionally intelligent woman, but she had been told that as a child, she did not begin to talk until age two, at which time she began to speak in full sentences. Her speech reflected thinking that was entirely abstracted from her emotions. Consistent with that information, she had a whole repertory of unusual gestures that we slowly realized were remnants of infantile preverbal affect and attitude expression. When she began to talk, she initially had no name for her mother. She believed she had had a loving relationship with her father, but through gradual understanding of various body sensations and gestures during the course of our sessions in response to her fears that I would attack her, she began to remember that her father had regularly sexually assaulted her.

She graduated from college with high honors, already having published papers in her field, and set her sights on actualizing the belief that she was smarter than almost everyone else and would become famous and that would make her feel good. However, when she began graduate school, she became suicidal, with auditory hallucinations and delusions, and was hospitalized. She saw the staff as her enemies and managed to get herself out of the hospital after some months by reconstituting her false self and doing such a good job pretending she was well that she apparently fooled the staff. She was able to complete her graduate degree and become a successful academic.

In the course of our work, Dorothy was initially extremely paranoid about me, assuming my personality was split between façade and secret reality (as was hers, without her realizing it) and that my real intentions were to sexually assault her. She knew nothing about her own emotions, especially rage and the desire to control others, and was largely unaware of body sensations. She "communicated" largely in a complex inadvertent repertory of gestures, the meaning of which we were slowly able to encode. Over the years, she gradually learned about her own hatred of humans, especially anyone who challenged her *modus operandi* as I did. She often confused her own thoughts and feelings with what she believed was going on with me. Her split mind was characterized by focusing on issues and pledges for a session or two, only to have them disappear from awareness for months or more. When I would remind her, she would get angry at me and accuse me of trying to distract her, as she was committed to dissociation as a way of being. The only way she could imagine intimacy was by programming everything that was to happen, scripting the man's actions so there was no room for a separate person. While she had major abstract abilities when it came to work, when it came to personal issues, she was very concrete, and when I tried to make an abstraction to aid understanding of what she was talking about, she was usually unable to understand it, another consequence of her success fragmenting aspects of her mind. She used her abstract abilities to separate herself from anything that might be personally or emotionally relevant.

We worked together for many years, during which she learned a great deal about her emotions, particularly the rage at human beings of which she had been unaware and her body sensations and their importance. She began to value her life and take better care of herself, developed some genuine though limited friendships, and found different work and some creative talents that were meaningful. However, we came to believe that after a final and unimaginably painful attempt to get her mother's attention very early in her life, she turned against further awareness of her feelings and turned away from human beings and that she was no longer able to make more than a friendship with another person.

Jacob

Jacob was almost 60 years of age when he was referred to me in the course of his search for yet another in a long series of therapists and psychoanalysts that had commenced in late adolescence. What turned out to be a search and destroy mission began after he had a brief hospitalization when an acute paranoid-delusional psychosis forced him to leave college. Jacob was unusually gifted, especially in mathematics and science, and he had done well at college for a time, until he became frightened that he was going to kill someone, told his father, who represented punitive authority in the family, and was hospitalized. After a short hospitalization, he returned to school, completed his studies, and began graduate school, but he became paralyzed and self-destructive trying to actualize a delusional conviction that he could solve what he believed was a legitimate mathematical problem, that of dividing by zero. His quest caused him to employ sophisticated mathematical reasoning in a self-destructive way so as to prevent him from actualizing what I came to realize were his significant mathematical talents.

Despite his crippling problems, Jacob was able to do well enough in the world of math- and physics-related technology to become a relatively high-level manager in a well-known electronics corporation.

When I met him many decades later, Jacob was a married father of three teenage sons. He complained of a sense of alienation from a world that he perceived as hostile and dangerous as well as of a literal sense of coldness that required him to wear an outdoor coat in my warm consulting room. Not long after we met, he took early retirement and for many years remained unemployed. Some years after commencing therapy with me, his wife, having become increasingly aware of his self-preoccupation and sadistic abuse of her, divorced him.

Since early adulthood, Jacob had been obsessively intent on making possessive relationships with women. Though he could not have put it into words, his goal in life, as it emerged from the stories he told me, seemed to be to get an erection through masturbation or intercourse, get into bed with a woman, and use it to gain control over the woman by discharging his sadism and bringing her to a point where she could not control herself and he had taken control of her identity and then somehow believe he had literally gotten inside her and was controlling her. It took many years to realize one aspect of this multi-determined pursuit was to avoid having to go out in the world, make a grown-up identity, and take care of himself. He was quite successful at seducing women and had a long history of exploiting masochistic women, who did not seem to have an independent identity of their own.

Jacob's problems, as we learned over the course of many years, revolved around his unresolved relationship with his mother. When he first came to see me, he was convinced that he loved her and that she had loved him, however a repetitive vivid set of images from various times in his childhood, articulated in photographic detail and clarity but without any emotional awareness, another story about her sadistic abuse and control of him. When I would attempt to articulate that story to him, he would turn on me viciously and imply I was crazy. She had told him as a child that his birth almost killed her. She undressed and dressed him in public even after he had reached puberty. She dressed him like a girl and physically controlled, invaded, and manipulated his body, primarily his anus, with her fingers and other devices. She treated him as though she believed he was seriously ill, although there was no evidence to substantiate this, and she had a group of doctors she called in regularly to examine, medicate, and restrict him. She would not let him play with other children but kept him in the house much of the time, particularly the bathroom and bedroom on the pretext that he was ill. She was seductive to him, taking him to bed with her and displaying herself to him in varying degrees of undress that excited him as a child and made him want to get under her skirts and inside her body through holes he believed existed, including one he imagined between her breasts. When father came home from work, mother would recite a litany of Jacob's badness and transgressions during the day, and father would beat him with a belt while mother looked on, wringing her hands in apparent dismay and crying. Needless to say, Jacob could never separate from his mother and any efforts to do so met with self-destruction. His identity, if one can call it that, was a mixture of enactment of self-destruction based on the way she had treated him and enactment of destruction toward others who tried to care about him that resembled how mother had treated him. Around age 7, he was playing ball with other boys in the street in defiance of mother's prohibition. The ball bounced in front of an oncoming car and Jacob, in a combination of what he retrospectively realized was an omnipotent sense he could fly and a simultaneous wish to kill himself and get it over with, dove in front of it, was hit and hospitalized for some days with a severe head injury.

In his later adolescent years, Jacob was haunted by powerful images of taking a knife and stabbing his mother to death, inhibited by reciprocal terrifying images of being apprehended and executed. While these images might seem inconsistent with his belief that he loved her, like his images she was invading and attacking him, they were unconnected with any emotional awareness of rage or any integrated sense of conflict. He experienced them as mysterious troubling obsessions. Having a knife became an important image in his adult life that he often had when talking to me, coming to signify the rage for which he had no emotional representation. He would keep himself from acting on his impulses by imagining himself being caught, convicted, and executed. He concretely confused the knife with his penis in intercourse, and it was associated with the urge to erect and ejaculate frequently and get it into women while believing he was controlling them. He and his wife had three children. He told me he had barely been able to restrain himself from pushing one of his children out of the carriage in an amusement park roller coaster when they were small.

Jacob presented to the world his cherished self-image as a know-it-all; a highly accomplished, highly intelligent, and cultured, mature man. He not only hid the fact he was in therapy from everyone, but he presented himself as being very knowledgeable in a therapist-like way about the problems of others, while he spent much of our sessions in a hostile, critical "analysis" of me and my multiple faults. Despite this façade, he lacked insight, knew nothing about his feelings, and acted impulsively and destructively without the slightest idea of what he was doing.

In the course of our work, his homicidal urges were at times quite direct and had a laser-like focus on me. For example, he had the urge to throw acid in my face when I greeted him or throw me downstairs as we said hello on the landing outside my office. Having had much experience with homicidal persons in hospital settings, I often sensed he was actually close to acting.

Although, as far as I could tell, Jacob was quite healthy, he was severely hypochondriacal; preoccupied with one after another real or imagined physical ailments that he was convinced were about to kill him and visits to doctors with whom he enacted these scenarios. He was preoccupied with his bowels and with his penis and its state of health and functional capacity to erect and ejaculate, around which his only sense of power seemed to revolve. He was addicted to pornography, and one of his favorite activities was masturbating to an image of a naked woman seated on his head with legs spread apart. He had a recurrent transient physical sensation that he had a woman's breast. It was so real that he made gestures with his hands to wipe it away. He made reflexive grimaces which he came to realize were efforts to imitate his mother's facial expressions, which he had actually practiced in front of a mirror during his childhood. One of his repetitive images was of me sitting in my own excrement. Another involved sadistically abusing my daughter. While these arose at meaningful places in our interaction, he had no awareness they represented rage and related ideas he was unable to express in mature language.

Jacob's lifelong quest for a therapist seemed to be a disguised quest for another victim he could control and destroy, not unlike his relationships with women. He had found several therapists who, like the women he seduced, were apparently reluctant to confront him and instead tended to placate him and comply with his various wishes rather than risk eliciting his vicious attacks. The single therapist who had begun to be of help, a person with an international reputation for success working with psychotic persons, had eventually terminated their relationship, explaining that Jacob was taxing some of his own personal areas of vulnerability more than he could constructively manage. In our relationship he talked nonstop. Efforts to intervene and give feedback were perceived as lethal assaults on his identity by a crazy man or monster, as evidence of my anger at him, or as evidence of how wrong or mistaken I was. He regularly distorted things I had said to him to fit this paradigm.

Despite his years of therapy prior to seeing me, Jacob was entirely unaware of the fact that he seemed to know only one way to interact, which we came to describe as kill or be killed. Consistent with his inability to differentiate us as separate persons, his behavior toward me was a mirror image of what he believed I was doing to him. He perceived himself as the victim, and it rapidly became evident he experienced me as trying to destroy his identity. He was full of images in which I was suffocating or strangling him, and he was being forced to "suck up" to me. For a time, he believed I was crazy and was overcome by images of me as a monster attacking him. At the same time, he believed his role as a patient was one of unrestrained license to vent his vicious hostility toward me and unending "analytic" litany of all my problems and failings, while expressing his grandiose beliefs about himself.

Beneath his grandiose omnipotent façade, however, was the truth Jacob fought for years against knowing; that he believed he was defective, that he felt powerless, frightened, and enraged, and that he did not feel he could survive without a woman who loved him unconditionally and acceded to his every wish. Over the course of many years of therapy, Jacob developed some insight, awareness of his thoughts and emotions, and control over himself. He stopped seeking out destructive merger states with women, took a more modest job, and began to live the semblance of an independent constructive life.

Lisabeth

Lisabeth's story is a bit different from that of Dorothy, who was blatantly and concretely destructive to herself, and of Jacob, who acted openly hateful and destructive toward others and was more subtly destructive to himself. It illustrates how disturbance in the attachment-separation phase of development leads to inability to develop a separate, coherent, purposeful sense of self and awareness of a separate other and to behavior that is destructive to one's life. Trauma in the attachment-separation phase does not always take the form of overt physical abuse, as it did in those two cases, so that from the perspective of an outside observer, a pathological family configuration might pass for normal, as it did in her case. Finally, it illustrates a remarkably successful productive false self.

Lisabeth was an attractive, intelligent, unmarried woman in her early 40s when she consulted me, complaining of intense anxiety bordering on panic that was compromising her ability to function. She had interrupted her increasingly successful career to go to graduate school, which she had almost completed. She asked for help to separate herself from an entanglement in a lesbian relationship in which she acted as surrogate parent for her partner's children. Many years previously, Lisabeth had been in a similar lesbian relationship and had undergone therapy that had concluded, in retrospect unsatisfactorily, with her being led to believe she was lesbian or bisexual, although she had always fled from any nascent engagement with a man and had never been able to achieve heterosexual intimacy.

Lisabeth's overt reluctance, one might even say terror, to form any kind of relationship with me was striking. Although she rapidly became very dependent on my absolute reliability and availability, her dread was manifest in the diarrhea she regularly experienced while waiting to see me, and that many years later we were able to translate into a complex of emotions that had remained somatic and never been mentally represented, including fear and rage. We first began to understand it as she became able to articulate her almost literal sense, she was excrement. She could barely sit still in the office. She avoided eye contact because it or any reference to a relationship with me literally sent a feeling of shock through her body. Early in our relationship when I made the retrospective mistake of asking her how she was feeling about me, she angrily admonished me, "don't you ever do that again!" My office was near the university she was attending, and paradoxically, she was obsessed with the desire to visualize me between sessions and tried to get glimpses through the window or when walking nearby. In those instances, when she would see me walking outside the office, she would flee in the other direction so I would not see her and we would not actually have to make contact.

This remarkable reluctance to acknowledge any kind of attachment seemed strikingly at odds with how stuck she claimed to be in the lesbian relationship from which she claimed she wanted my help to extricate herself. Nonetheless, it was not long before she was able to end it without much specific work on the issue in therapy. The paradox resolved itself when it gradually became apparent, she was developing a similar all-consuming adhesive attachment to me, in which she strived to believe we were not separate. She would shadow or stalk me between appointments, staring up at the window of my office, or she would drive by my house and sometimes lurk in the neighborhood hoping for a glimpse of me through the window. She became catastrophically panicked and angry over any separation from me or indeed, any indication I had a separate life and loves of my own that did not include her. She was remarkably attuned to and searched out any details she could find about my life and used them to rationalize the belief, associated with intense anger, that I had a perfect existence from which she was excluded. She imagined that I had no needs and "had it all," for I experienced only good feelings and the love and adulation of everyone, a state she strived to attain that we eventually recognized as narcotic or death-like. Even the idea that I needed money for my work was difficult for her to comprehend, so she resented having to pay me. She believed that she was just an object of my therapeutic technique, and that when we were out of sight, she was totally absent from my thoughts and caring. During even brief periods of separation, she experienced a cataclysmic sense of personal annihilation. During one separation early in our relationship, she became panicked and experienced her arms as having been amputated. In essence, in order for her to survive, she believed I had to become her and she, me. Over time, we realized she was treating me as though I were her mother, from whom she was unable to separate.

While one would expect another person to feel better when she said she felt better, Lisabeth said she felt worse. She had been taught that having caring feelings and making attachments to people and things was wrong, and it was a sign of selfishness, feeling "too good" about oneself. So, she reflexively destroyed such nascent feelings about me.

One might conclude from this description that Lisabeth was not very bright and led a regressed disorganized life. Far from it. As our work continued, she finished graduate school and launched a career in education in which she was in charge of a large organization, respected and admired for her organizational and human relations skills and her innovative creativity. However, none of this was integrated with her emotional life, which was a secret she shared only with me. Another paradox was that as she was more and more successful professionally, she became increasingly terrified, even paranoid, that the people with whom she worked would find out the "truth" about what worthless excrement she was.

How did all this come about? Mother had a full-time career as human relations expert. As a baby, Lisabeth was largely raised by a nanny as mother was busy with her career. Subsequently, she spent much time with her maternal grandmother who came to live with them after her parents divorced when she was 5. Lisabeth recalls many subsequent occasions when mother would complain what a burden it was to be abandoned by her husband and left with the care of two children. She could not recall being held or hugged, but did recall a sense of repulsion at being close to her mother's body. As a child, she had few friends and preferred to spend time hiding out in the basement of their house or wandering in the fields and woods hear her house where she was fascinated with small animals, reptiles, and insects, that she liked to "capture" and take care of and with whom she seemed to identify.

After her parents divorced, Lisabeth's mother led her to believe her father was a weak man who had been seduced by an evil woman and that her father had a new family and would no longer recognize her as his daughter. Many years later, Lisabeth discovered that mother had used legal means to prevent him from having much contact with her, and he was too passive to protest much. Mother never formed another relationship. When Lisabeth made ambivalent attempts to form relationships with persons outside the core family, mother always used her analytic "skill" to point out their various faults and caution her against getting involved.

After her father left, Lisabeth began to have tantrums and mother took her to see a child therapist. She learned many years later that they believed she was angry at her father for leaving. She and her mother initiated a game in which Lisabeth was in a chair with a spoked back that looked like a cage and told to roar like a lion.

Lisabeth, her older brother, and her mother formed a tight unit, more or less immune from outside influence, which presented an image of normalcy to the world, and derived meaning from mother's belief system. Mother conveyed the sense that she knew everything. She told the children she spoke Greek and was an expert on Greek mythology, and though she never demonstrated such knowledge, she was almost literally a Greek god to Lisabeth. What Lisabeth repeated to me of what seemed like mother's stereotypic repetitive statements and maxims appeared ordinary enough in formal content, but in the context and tone in which she said them, as imitated by Lisabeth, they seemed like disguised judgments, criticisms, and instructions about how to think and behave. Most important was not to care deeply about anyone outside the family either because there was something wrong with them or because one should remember one's heritage and not feel "too dependent." For much of our relationship, Lisabeth would counter my comments with contrary sayings or "interpretations" quoted from her mother about her, others, and the world. Lisabeth had become her mother's most effective propaganda minister, discouraging anyone who might begin to raise critical questions, as she did with me during our early years when I would try to clarify some of the implications of things she told me.

Lisabeth quoted the professional jargon mother used, to interpret to her children the disqualifying problems of anyone Lisabeth might begin to show interest in, making comments such as "why do you have a need to feel that way?" Or "I'm keeping an eye on that relationship; I have some doubts about her." Early in our relationship, mother advised Lisabeth to remember her heritage and not become too dependent on me, and she told Lisabeth to dismiss any caring feelings she might have as "just transference," meaning they were not real. Lisabeth reflexively attacked her nascent feelings, leading to a habit of fleeing from anyone who began to arouse them. As a result, she did not allow herself to have strong emotions and she had no names for her feelings, manifesting instead the intense anxiety that resulted from their somatic precursors combined with her attacks on them. She regularly "consulted" with mother about potential friends in an unconscious effort to help her suppress any nascent attachment. In her early forties, when I met her, Lisabeth still spent most of her vacation time with her mother and brother, who was even more crippled in the realm of having an independent life than Lisabeth. She considered her brother her best friend, despite his history of openly abusive treatment of her. Shortly after meeting me, she told me her brother was the most handsome man she knew, far more attractive than me, so that when she eventually showed me a photo of him and he looked very ordinary, it came as a shock.

As she grew, Lisabeth developed her own false self-social façade like that of her mother, as well as athletic skills and adventurousness based on what subsequently turned out to be dangerous risk-taking motivated by a combination of her sense of worthlessness or defectiveness, an unawareness of feelings of fear, and her learned way of getting the attention of a mother who did not seem to care for her otherwise, but was a mental health professional who seemed to get satisfaction with finding things wrong with other people. She developed a belief that, which was based on fact, she could do many physical and mechanical things better than most men, and when she first came to see me, it turned out she actually believed she had a tiny penis. She was quite attractive and intelligent, and men were very interested in her, but once they showed it, she fled from them in nameless terror.

It turned out that she believed that it was her job as patient to continue to be a problem to me, for after all, as a psychoanalyst, I "needed" patients with something the matter with them. It followed that if she felt "too good" about herself, it would lead to an end to her therapy as I would have no more interest in her, and as she experienced it, she would no longer exist. Mention of the word "termination" elicited a cataclysmic electric-current-like body-mind end of the world reaction that we discovered meant extinction; the end of her world as she understood it. Her reaction was so intense, physical, and disruptive that it was a long time before the word termination could even be mentioned and its usual meaning in a therapeutic context talked about.

Over the course of many years, Lisabeth came to understand more about herself and to feel anger and separation between herself and a mother she realized not only had not wanted and loved her but had used her as a repository for mother's own low self-esteem, rejection, and rage. She realized that her aversion to emotional awareness was related to her low self-esteem and her lack of a separate sense of identity. Late in life, she was able to form a relationship with and then marry a kind intelligent man who did not pose a threat to her as he was rather passive and did not have a strong sense of identity of his own and did not manifest strong emotions. She was able to tolerate increasing awareness of separation and difference from me. But she continued to struggle with self-esteem and to remain attracted to the state of regression her mother had encouraged as a way of avoiding the work of bearing and orienting herself around her emotions and making an independent life for herself.

Charles

Charles was in his late 20s when he consulted me. He was living a withdrawn reclusive existence, supported by a family fortune he had inherited from a several generation family business run by his father who had committed suicide in Charles's early teens. He was immobilized by a sense of paranoid hopelessness in a world he believed to be hostile and dangerous, and seriously contemplated suicide. He spent much of his time in the basement of his apartment engaged in repetitive behavior, taking apart, cleaning, and rebuilding his precious motorcycle. After many years, we came to realize that he was repeating a destructive entanglement with his mother that he could not thoughtfully understand and move beyond and that he seemed to reenact in every phase of his life. The skill it took to do the motorcycle work turned out to be a precursor of one of the strengths that he was able to develop over the years, a remarkable capacity to build or repair almost anything in the non-human sphere, from houses and furniture to sophisticated electrical and electronic gear, and to create art. But it also presaged another of his characteristics, as his activities turned out to represent endless repetitions of sadomasochistic identity-devastating interactions with his psychotic mother. Not long after he began seeing me, he got drunk one night and held a shotgun to his head, but at the last minute he decided to call me and ask for help. The "help" he seemed to be looking for was another venue for endless repetition of rage-discharging sequences.

One of the common features of the backgrounds of the people whose stories I am recounting (and other instances of psychosis) is that the family environments of their childhood were encapsulated, like cults, isolated from feedback or input. They presented sufficiently normal facades so as not to attract unusual attention from the outside world. Charles's childhood was spent in relative isolation in the country home of his wealthy upper-class parents and their servants. His mother was an out of control, probably psychotic, alcoholic woman who, judging from her behavior, was filled with rage and hatred, especially of males. Her daily routine consisted of getting drunk and verbally and sometimes physically assaulting Charles' father during the times he could not evade her presence. At night, father would lock himself in his bedroom or retreat to another house on the family estate, leaving Charles and his brother alone with mother, who prowled the halls, banging on the locked door of father's bedroom when he was there, and alternately invading the bedrooms of Charles or his older brother, which had no locks. She would climb into bed with Charles and rain name-calling assaults down on him while telling him how special he was and pleading for his love. He would try his best not to move and to withdraw and shut down his mind, like a cornered animal playing dead. He turned the rage he could not express to her inward on his mind and into his undifferentiated conviction the world was a hostile place. Eventually, mother would roll over facing away from him and fall into a drunken stupor, often with her nightgown hiked up so that Charles was confronted with her naked buttocks. In the morning, the kitchen and bathroom would stink of vomit and diarrhea, and while mother slept it off, Charles would try his best to clean up the mess, get her some breakfast, and get ready for school.

Father was as reclusive and withdrawn as Charles turned out to be. He commuted to work as the CEO of the successful multigeneration family business and often took trips. He absented himself during mother's drunken tirades and abandoned Charles and his brother to their mother's mercy. He did make some efforts to get good schooling for his son and encourage him in that area as well as in sports, but Charles and his father had no emotional bond and the efforts felt mechanical. Charles was passive, and while he tried to comply with father's expectations, the world mystified and terrified him. He came to depend on being the special focus of his mother's attentions, and he lived out a kind of perverse Oedipal fantasy that involved rejection of his father and a bizarre sense of incestuous control of his mother. He constructed a delusion, amalgamating the belief she would be changed the next time he saw her and all the problems would somehow be taken away, with an undifferentiated idea of retaliation that involved withholding and attacking his own mind in the face of her pleas to love her that she made while abusing him. Charles barely got by at school. His withdrawal and problems reading and writing were understood by the family to be the product of a genetic learning disability, for which we found no evidence whatsoever.

Around the time Charles entered puberty, father was hospitalized for "depression" at a "retreat" known mostly for "drying out" wealthy alcoholics. It is not clear what treatment he got, if any, but he was eventually discharged and, it seems in retrospect, sent home to die. He took to his bed, where he spent the days more or less immobilized and alone. Soon thereafter, Charles was sent to boarding school. In Charles's early adolescence, father shot himself in the head with a pistol, leaving Charles feeling utterly hopeless and alone with his mother and the family fortune.

Our relationship was characterized by Charles's passivity and withholding. His sessions consisted of prolonged silences, during which Charles would breathe audibly and rhythmically through his mouth in a kind of snorting manner that reminded me of a steam engine while darting glances at me and then looking away. When I asked him to share his thoughts, he would claim his mind was blank. Over a long period of time, we gradually discovered his *modus operandi* was a process of passive angry withholding from others while attacking the contents of his mind so as to effectively psychically annihilate himself and the other person. His inner experience was not of formed thoughts, but of somatic tension in various parts of his body along with sadomasochistic images like chopping wood or chopping himself to pieces that, for a long time, he had no words to express. His mental state with me was a repetition of the experiences with his mother that had never been elevated to the realm of thoughtful reflection. He was convinced that my efforts to pay attention to him and encourage him to talk were a combination of hostile attacks and encouragements for him to enact rageful attacks of his own. Our work was made especially difficult as although he had almost no life of his own, he could live without working because of his inheritance and he claimed that he was fine other than the way he behaved with me. I came to think that he was using me as a kind of dissociated toilet, as his mother had used him.

During the many difficult years of our work, Charles gradually gained some ability to think and to use language to describe his thoughts; abilities he was convinced he did not have prior to therapy. Very gradually, his sense of undifferentiation from a world he experienced as a terrible place filled with hostile people emerged, and even more slowly awareness of enormous rage and passive sense of entitlement, not just to have his traumatic childhood made up to him, but delusionally to have someone make it never have happened, a task he had unwittingly been attempting to do by attacking his mental contents.

Charles was not able to initiate and follow through with goals of his own or to make a career for himself, despite his considerable ability. It turned out that he had considerable artistic talent, and in the course of our work, he began to create installations that used old home movies, often of women, and involved hypnotic repetition of images. They were made in a darkened studio and displayed in dark rooms. His creations got notice from the art community and even significant museum recognition, but when he realized that this was yet another repetition of the repetitive reenactment of his destructive sadomasochistic relationship with his mother, he stopped making them. Some years later, he began to express himself in other media, and while his work was quite interesting, he could not actively organize himself and engage with others sufficiently to display and sell it and make a career.

He had serial relationships with women with large breasts with whom he enacted in muted form what he had been unable to do with his mother, using his penis as a way to discharge rage without awareness of what he was doing, while having simultaneous fantasies that his suckling behavior was erasing his past. Unlike Jacob, he was not actively harmful to others, and he picked women who were also withdrawn and had problems making mature relationships but seemed to find his sexuality exciting.

Charles eventually married, but his wife was unable to get pregnant. With great ambivalence, Charles decided to adopt. The marriage gradually deteriorated and ended in divorce during the first years of his son's life, as he and his wife became more aware of their mutual withdrawal and hostility. At first, he was psychologically merged with the baby, its helplessness, and the fantasy that the baby might be disabled and be unable or unwilling to grow. But his son became the love of his life; the best thing that ever happened to him. Surprisingly, he became a good caring father, concerned that his son gets what he had not received from parents. But he remained alone and unable to make a separate relationship with a woman, despite feelings of loneliness.

President Donald Trump

Psychoanalysts have often speculated about the psychology of persons who commit acts of overt destruction toward others, like mass shootings, or bombings, or horrific murders, but we rarely have the opportunity to analyze such individuals in depth, and when we do have the opportunity to interview them, their hostility and mistrust of others and the compulsory, involuntary situation in which they come to mental health attention, usually a pretrial evaluation or a treatment that is mandated as part of their sentence, is hardly conducive to the trust and openness necessary to produce the kind of in-depth information that requires collaboration between analyst and patient.

The former President of the United States, Donald Trump, has been overtly destructive to others in a myriad of ways by a consensus of educated observers. Whether he has been destructive to himself as well or whether in light of his early history of being the helpless victim of neglect his social success controlling and being destructive to others might be considered adaptive and at least for him, constructive, the reader can judge after reading what is known of his story.

Trump has left a remarkable and detailed trail of oral history supplemented by media accounts and accounts from those close to him, which, taken together, provide a substantial window into his personality and the way his mind works. Every issue and encounter is reduced to whether he is right and great, and he makes and incites others to make violent verbal and behavioral attacks on those who differ with him or he perceives as different from him, who are perceived as lethal threats. He seems unaware of the meaning of such concepts as truth, coherence, or consistency, and he regularly contradicts himself, all in the service of maintaining the sense that he is the sole arbiter of what is real and true. No matter how it may seem to others. And he has enjoyed remarkable success assembling followers who seem to agree with him by appealing to their desire for power and for license to enact their own hostility. He rejects education, science, and any discipline based on independent critical thinking and makes it clear he believes he knows more and better than anyone else. His capacity to deny and distort facts and consensual reality, for example that he was soundly defeated in a fairly conducted presidential election, meets the criteria for delusional thinking. Shortly after he lost the election, the *Washington Post* compiled a list of false claims he made and lies he told during his presidency that numbered more than 30,000. And the things he accuses others of are usually acts of deception and hostility that might well be accounts of things he does himself but either denies or believes are reasonable, indicating difficulty differentiating self from other. In her recent book, *Confidence Man* (2022), Maggie Haberman points out his difficulty understanding time; his tendency to live in the present moment while reflecting grievances and self-preoccupation related to his past.

Trump exemplifies the destruction a human being in a position of power can wreak on others, on society, and even on the environment and the human species. Hardly a day goes by without him not only calling people whom he believes are different from him names and encouraging others to join with him in so doing, but in enacting dangerous attacks on them as well.

During the 2016 election campaign, he did not content himself with disagreeing with his opponent Hillary Clinton; he portrayed her as evil and criminal. He was not being metaphorical; he called her a criminal and encouraged his followers at rallies to chant "jail her, lock her up" and pick fights with her supporters, reminiscent of lynch mob behavior. And he did everything he could to have her investigated for crimes there was no objective evidence she had committed. Some of the "crimes" he accused her of, related to Russia and to collusion with big business, were actually things there was abundant evidence he himself was guilty of but denied.

In a July 2015 pronouncement, Trump, who avoided the draft during the Vietnam War by claiming bone spurs in his foot that there is no evidence he actually has, attacked Senator John McCain, generally acclaimed as a hero for his service flying combat missions in that war, saying in a statement remarkable for its contradictions, "He's not a war hero. He's a war hero because he was captured. I like people who weren't captured."

He claimed that the marriage of his political rival Elizabeth Warren was a "phony, disgusting deal," while dismissing as false significant evidence not only that he had numerous extramarital affairs but that he has repeatedly used his position of power to exploit and sexually abuse women and has boasted of his success being able to fondle their bodies at will.

In a speech to Jews at the Israeli-American Council on December 8, 2019, Trump, who regularly boasted what a wonderful man he is, despite well-documented behavior toward others in ruthless pursuit of the aggrandizement of his own real estate empire, said "A lot of you are in the real estate business because I know you very well, you're brutal killers, not nice people at all."

As President, he revoked previous policies and legislation designed to protect against international, social, and individual destructiveness and destruction of the natural environment.

Trump has made relentless efforts to destroy the constitutionally mandated balance of power, separation, and independence of the legislative and judiciary branches of government, and to bring them under his control. He makes no secret of his belief that members of the judicial branch and people with authority to tally election results should do his bidding. At one point, he stated that perhaps the Constitution ought to be revised as it didn't reflect his beliefs.

Trump is not typical of persons who by general social consensus are labeled destructive, however, insofar as he has attained great social power and a loyal base of followers who remain committed to him no matter what he says or does. Early in his first election campaign, he boasted in a tweet that he could step outside his office onto Fifth Avenue and shoot someone and his followers would believe his actions justified and reasonable. His subsequent behavior and its consequences, at least at the time of this writing, have done nothing to cast doubt on his belief. His wealthy privileged upbringing, his ability to use his money and power to manipulate and control the law in his favor, and his cleverness in enlisting a loyal following who do not question him no matter what he does and says, have enabled him to do more or less whatever he wants. In addition to self-satisfaction, he has enjoyed remarkable financial, social, sexual, and political success. Almost half the population think he is not just normal, but exceptional – and perhaps he is.

I want to make clear that I am not making a diagnosis of the former president, even though his inclusion in this chapter that predominantly exemplifies psychosis might suggest otherwise. During the presidential campaign, there was a heated controversy about whether mental health professionals are qualified, ethically entitled, and publicly responsible to make diagnostic or analytic statements about public figures. The tendency of some psychoanalysts and psychiatrists to do this is an unfortunate legacy of the behavior of Sigmund Freud, who made diagnostic and analytic pronouncements about colleagues who questioned his authority. His lamentable tendency extended into the public sphere when he collaborated with William Bullitt during the early years of Nazism on a biography of Woodrow Wilson, whom he had neither met nor examined. He attributed Wilson's signing of the Treaty of Versailles to his putative neurosis. I believe it is unethical to use one's professional authority and competence to diagnose someone who has not asked for help and whom the analyst has not had the opportunity to professionally evaluate. The motivation usually derives from critical feelings and helplessness to bring about change and is not based on the therapeutic good of the person. It is a disguised expression of value judgment and name-calling that suggests retaliation in kind for some of Trump's own behavior.

What can be said, beyond that the former President has been very destructive, is that his behavior and mentation, as illustrated from news reports and numerous quoted comments, are consistent with a description of primordial mentation. The purpose of this chapter is to illustrate how maladaptive persistence of primordial mentation due to failures in the attachment-separation phase of development leads to individual destructiveness in adulthood, so the Trump example is not clear, as it is an admixture of destruction and unusual adaptation.

Briefly, to recapitulate the characteristic of primordial mentation, they include inability to distinguish others as separate individuals from oneself and a tendency to animate them with characteristics and feelings that objectively belong to the self. They include the tendency to enact one's mental content rather than think reflectively about it and control it internally. It is rooted in body sensations and perceptions and behavior rather than identification and control of one's emotions and related thoughts. It is concrete rather than symbolic and metaphoric. It is not integrated into a coherent narrative but allows for inconsistencies and contradictions. It does not distinguish time, past from present and from an imagined future. In short, it reflects a belief system rather than a flexible thoughtful adaptation to consensual reality.

During the final apocalyptic destructive phase of his presidency, Trump gave a speech to his followers in which he incited them to invade the Capitol, the literal and symbolic seat of government, assault the legislators within who were about to certify the Electoral College vote confirming without doubt his loss to Biden in the election, and kill the Vice President who had refused his bidding to falsify the results of the election. Here are some excerpts from his inflammatory speech to his followers on January 6, 2020. His confusion between self and other is evident, and not just oratorical:

> **We will never give up**. We will never concede. It doesn't happen. You don't concede when there's theft involved. Our country has had enough. **We will not take it anymore, and that is what this is all about.** And to use a favorite term that all of you people really came up with, **we will stop the steal....** Republicans are constantly **fighting like a boxer with his hands tied behind his back**. It's like a boxer. And we want to be so nice. We want to be so respectful of everybody, including **bad peopl**e. And we're going to have to **fight much harde**r. We're going to walk down to the Capitol, and we're going to cheer on our brave senators and congressmen and women,

and we're probably not going to be cheering so much for some of them, because you'll never take back our country with weakness. **You have to show strength**, and you have to be strong.

This rambling soliloquy is remarkable not only as an illustration of his destructiveness, but for the complete confusion and undifferentiation between self and other, subject and object, and about who is doing or is to do what to whom, which I turn to next. This same man told an audience at a political rally that he had been cheated of the Nobel Peace Prize!

Trump is concrete and action oriented. He openly disparages science. During the COVID-19 pandemic and in relation to global warming, he dismissed scientists and their findings, claimed that he is a genius who follows the truth that his "gut" tells him, and even advocated things like drinking bleach to kill the virus, at the same time that when he contracted the illness himself, he demanded and expected the best medicines available.

Pronoun confusions and interchangeability of the realms of imagination and reality often occur around the second year of life. While even small infants quickly learn to make functional distinctions between important persons, they struggle psychologically to distinguish the worlds of imagination and reality, to distinguish their separate selves from the selves of others, and to distinguish the use of words as symbols and metaphors from their concrete use as things of action. Slogans like "sticks and stones will break my bones, but names will never hurt me" come from the period in which the child is learning that names are just thoughts, symbols, and ideas. Most of us learn to recognize the difference between the word and the object, to respect the differences of others so long as they are not directly trying to hurt us, to recognize the difference between our wishes and reality, and we come to express anger in discourse without throwing epithets as though they were things. Trump did not.

Consider Trump's habitual misuse of pronouns and his readiness to call others derogatory names. At an award ceremony for Native Americans who served as code breakers in WWII, for example, he stated, "We have a representative in Congress who they say was here a long time ago. They call her Pocahontas. But you know what, I like you." As it was Trump who used "Pocahontas" as a derogatory epithet for Elizabeth Warren, we would expect to hear a subjective "I" to acknowledge his authorship, but instead he speaks as an undifferentiated "we" and "they." His concluding "I" is consistent with his failure to take ownership of the epithet demeaning Native Americans he used only seconds before. He regularly refers to the author of actions he has taken or intends to take by presidential decree as "we." And he frequently refers to "Donald Trump" as though he were someone else referring to him, the way mothers refer to their children early in development.

For example, he tweeted that the "Trump/Russia story was an excuse used by the Democrats as justification for losing the election. Perhaps Trump just ran a great campaign?"

Material about Trump's childhood that might help us understand his apparent developmental difficulties during the attachment-separation phase of infant development is sparse. He is closed about his childhood, as with all details of his personal life other than occasional expressions of admiration for his father and a kind of pride in the evolution of their relationship from one of hostility and defiance to one in which he came to act much like father and got father's support for doing so. He has little to say about his mother or the rest of the family. He has used legal means along with his enormous wealth to extract non-disclosure agreements from women including his first wife and suppress whatever information they might have. Until recently, the 2015 history of the Trump dynasty by Gwenda Blair, sparse on Trump's life as it is and lacking in information about how she documented what she wrote, has been the most complete source of information. In 2020, Trump's niece Mary Trump published a more detailed account in defiance of one of his numerous non-disclosure agreements and despite legal attempts by Trump and other family members to block publication. Most of what follows comes from her biography, which is consistent with what little was previously known.

Although niece Mary is a clinical psychologist with an excellent reputation, it must be noted that she is hardly an unbiased objective biographer. Mary obviously dislikes her uncle, and much of what she writes about Trump's childhood probably came from her father Fred Junior, Trump's older brother. He had reason for animosity as he was openly denigrated and mistreated by their father Fred Sr. and by Donald. Fred Jr. was the only sibling who tried to separate himself from the undifferentiated family identity and literally fly the coop (he became an airline pilot). His effort aborted tragically with death from alcoholism at age 42. On the other hand, to balance the scales of justice somewhat, Mary's effort to separate from the family has involved trying to understand it and has led to her becoming a respected clinical psychologist.

Trump's mother Mary was the youngest of ten children. She came to the United States at age 18 from the Scottish Hebrides, now the site of one of his golf courses whose importance Trump regularly brags about. She became a domestic in the mansion of Andrew Carnegie in New York, where at age 24 she met her future husband, Fred Sr., then a rising financial magnate.

Trump's mother is described by Trump's niece as a self-centered unpredictable woman who tried to use her children to make her feel good and was largely unaware of and attentive to their needs as separate persons. This fits Mary Ainsworth's (1983) description in Chapter 13 of rejecting mothers and their anxious-avoidant infants.

Mary had five children, two girls and three boys, of whom Donald was number four. Maryanne, the eldest sibling, is almost 9 years older than Donald. Fred Jr., the next oldest was 7 ½ years older than Donald. There was a 4 ½ year hiatus between Elizabeth, the second sister, and Donald. Mary was advised by her doctors not to have more children after Donald, but when he was around 1 ½ years of age, presumably at the height of the attachment-separation phase, mother became pregnant with her last child, Trump's younger brother Robert. Robert was born when Donald was about 2 years and 2 months of age. About 9 months after Robert's birth, when Donald would have been less than 3, mother suffered a sudden life-threatening hemorrhage that required emergency hysterectomy and ovariectomy. Her life hung in the balance for a time, and what mothering Donald had experienced seems to have vanished thereafter. In the year that followed, mother developed septicemia and required several additional surgeries. She developed severe osteoporosis as a consequence of removal of her ovaries. She was apparently accident prone, and as a result of osteoporosis, she had frequent fractures subsequent to the surgery. She developed insomnia and nocturnal wanderings as well; a characteristic Donald Trump also displays. Donald's care subsequent to her illnesses seems to have been divided between maids and his sister Maryanne, who was 12 at the time mother was hospitalized.

Information about Father Fred, about whom more is known, has been saved for last, although his in-your-face hostility, much like that of his son, overshadows mother's much less conspicuous but probably more profound influence. The basic damage to Donald was almost certainly done before father administered the *coup de grace*. Father seems to have been a self-centered liar; an uncaring, sexist male who was verbally abusive to others, including his children, and was an expert at manipulating others in order to get what he wanted without regard to truth or scruples. He was an autocrat at home but was basically absent and preoccupied with his astronomically successful real estate career. Father was contemptuous of Donald's older brother Fred and encouraged Donald to join in ridiculing him. The failure to appreciate the separateness of others and requirement that others be clones of oneself is another characteristic shared by father and son. Donald's growing nasty defiant behavior presented a problem for father. Both within the family and at school, Donald soon became out of control and socially incorrigible.

By the time Donald was 12, his elder brother Fred Jr. had labeled him "the great I am," an eerie echo of Trump's more recent statement that he is "a stable genius." Donald had become like father and acted contemptuous of outside authority. By age 13, no one could control him. Donald openly defied his mother, bullied his younger brother, was contemptuous of his older one, and was rebellious and out of control at school. Finally, father, who was on the school board, acceded to suggestions of others, and had him sent to a military boarding school.

The rest, as they say, is history. It is remarkable how Trump has been able to use his mind and behavior to compensate for deficits in his early upbringing, for example, by using his power to control women, even boasting about his success publicly manipulating women's bodies whenever he chooses. He has managed to become the center of everyone's attention and actualize his delusional belief that he is the greatest at everything he undertakes. Only two weeks after revealing he had what apparently was a severe case of COVID-19 and required an extraordinary combination of drugs in order to survive, he dismissed the severity of his illness and actually claimed that he felt "like Superman." Once at the mercy of the leaders of the military school to which he was sent as an adolescent and presumably disciplined by its military leaders, as president he has not only demonstrated his reverence for the military, in his role as Commander-in-Chief he stocked his administration with high-ranking military. Though the relationships began as glowing honeymoons, once his picks showed evidence of having minds of their own, he capriciously turned on most of them and fired them.

Donald Trump and Sigmund Freud: Strange bedfellows

Before turning from the topic of individual destructiveness to its reiteration and translation into the social system, I should like to juxtapose the story of Donald Trump with that of Sigmund Freud. At first glance, such a contrast may seem to make no sense, as the effect of these two men on our social systems and on civilization as a whole could hardly be more dissimilar. Judging from the admittedly limited information available, however, there are remarkable similarities between the childhoods of the two men that make their equally striking differences even more amazing. Little is known about both their early childhoods, which may say something about their relationships with their mothers, but each apparently sustained trauma, inconsistency, and insecurity in the attachment-separation phase. While each has had little to say about his mother, each has been articulate about the importance of his father in particular and male authority in general. Here, the similarity ends and we are left to speculate about the divergence of their respective lives and influence on society. Trump has been one of the most destructive forces in recent history, whereas Freud's study of the human mind led to the creation of a new psychological discipline; one based on a theory about paternal authority and presumed developments subsequent to the phase of attachment and separation.

How are we to account for the striking difference? Much of it may relate to a difference in their mothering experience. Both mothers appear to have been narcissistic. But as far as we know, Trump's mother had very little interest in him, whereas Freud was very important to his mother. His specialness, however, came at a cost. She demanded exceptional responsibility from him, although it appears to have been based not so much on caring about him as a separate person as on her own narcissistic expectations of what he should do. Differences in their respective fathers may have played a part, as well. Freud's father, though not very accomplished, appears to have been mild-mannered and friendly, whereas Trump's father modeled and rewarded ruthless self-aggrandizing behavior and encouraged enactment of his son's hostility.

16

SOCIAL DESTRUCTIVENESS

The clash between groups: Belief versus belief, belief versus reflective thought, and reflective thought versus reflective thought

Chapter 8 describes the primordial mental process that humans share with members of other species and the reflective representational thought that is unique to homo sapiens. The origins of reflective representational thought were traced to the lengthy period of maturation that occurs after birth that is unique to humans, and the learned acquisition, elaboration, and intergenerational transmission of knowledge necessitated and enabled by prolonged dependency on caregivers during that time. Chapter 12 describes how the resulting evolution of mind has led to a corresponding evolution of human social organization from one based on social sharing of primordial mentation, in which the individual person is subsumed as a component part of the group to one based on the primacy and rights of each member as a separate reflective person.

Just as not all individuals are able to separate and become mature reflective thinkers, so society includes groupings organized for the most part on undifferentiated primordial mentation and others based for the most part on reflective thought and the choices that enables. One result of this polarization is recurrent conflicts between organizations based on reflective thought and others based on shared belief systems. However, like groups also clash. Conflicts among groups organized around competing belief systems are commonplace, and persons engaged in reflective thought can reach conflicting conclusions and form groups in opposition to one another. The more extreme forms of social conflict this chapter focuses on range from outright criminal behavior to varying degrees of political upheaval, and include cults and movements organized around radical belief systems that promote violence, as well as conflicts between governments based on dictatorship and fascism and ones that are more democratic.

DOI: 10.4324/9781003442318-16

Our first experience of a social organization consists of childhood immersion in whatever system provides us with life-sustaining food, shelter, and a modicum of purposeful organization. Many are not fortunate enough to have a nuclear family or to have an experience beyond loveless instrumental survival. This initial organization serves as a mental template for formation and membership in the larger social organizations that are a part of adult life. Another way to say it is that these organizations, of which the family is the most "normal" example, comprise our first group.

One remarkable difference between the human species and other animals, including our primate ancestors, is that most other species rear their young in intact biologically programmed family structures typical for the species in the relatively short period of time required between birth and functional independence. The biology of neoteny in homo sapiens by contrast has led to individual and social human differences in parenting and child-rearing during the relatively lengthy period of maturation subsequent to birth that lead to idiosyncratic learning experiences that transmit, intergenerationally, similar experiences that parents had as children.

Not only is the family – or whatever has come to substitute for it due to the vicissitudes of human learning – our first experience in a social group, the experience comes at a time when infants and small children view themselves and the world through the lens of primordial mind, are not psychologically differentiated from others, and the elements of proto-self that are not differentiated have yet to be integrated into a separate individual sense of self. In other words, the original group is a shared belief system for reasons that are psychological as well as practical. One of the most profound thinkers about the nature of groups was Wilfred Bion (*Experiences in Groups*, 1961). He writes that the primordial mental organization that characterizes groups "is one in which physical and psychological are as yet undifferentiated" (1951, p. 103).

Infants ordinarily emerge from this primordial group mentality and the lengthy period of extrauterine maturation by acquiring a second reflective thoughtful mental process and a separate sense of self, including the capacity to make independent choices, even when at the same time choosing to be members of groups that have an element of shared belief. Mature persons are by nature simultaneously rugged individuals and committed groupies. However, when the original sustaining environment is unable to provide the secure consistent holding necessary for such development and flexibility but enforces forms of compliance rather than encouraging growth and individuation, the family is no longer a nest that encourages growth and development of the capacity to selectively choose between individual and group mentality. Instead, it might be thought of as the first cult. The cases in the preceding chapter are examples. Lisabeth even came in the course of her analysis to refer to the organization comprising herself, her brother, and their mother as a cult.

Social organizations that are based on shared primordial mentation and can be characterized as shared belief systems are not always destructive. Many are basically peaceful and harmonious, though insular. They do not encourage acquisition of reflective thought as part of child development and view its manifestations including education and science as dangerous as they encourage questions about belief systems that are often couched in religious authoritarian right and wrong terms. Parents and children have loving relationships so long as there is no deviation. As for the organizations themselves, so long as they are not disturbed by outside influences based on reflective thought and its consequences, all remains well. They are conservative in the sense of being predicated on conformity, and not promoting the education and encouragement necessary for separation and development of a self that is organized around reflective thought and respect for individual differences. Social destructiveness occurs when members of such groups become "contaminated" by rational thought, science, logic, and appreciation of differences, either in the form of rebellion of individual members or of contact and conflict with groups based on reflective thought. The so-called Scopes Monkey Trial, an example of such a clash, is described later in the chapter.

Turning to inherently destructive social systems and social conflicts, cults are the most malignant examples. Cults are systems comprised of two types of persons who basically share primordial mental activity and are hostile to reflective thought and individual difference. Passive compliant followers and an active pontifical leader share a common identity based on primordial mentation that is manifestly delusional. They license and encourage violent expression of unintegrated, undifferentiated, uncontrolled rage. Neither party is able to develop and sustain an integrated cohesive internal mind and to separate and live without the other in a world that values reflective thought and individual differences. Specifically, members of cults are unable to experience, reflect upon, and control emotions, particularly fear and rage. Such persons enact these aspects of self that they are unable to own, as though they are reactions to characteristics of others. In other words, they tend to be paranoid and attribute the rage and malevolent intentions they are unaware of within themselves to others. Examples include Charles Manson and his followers, who murdered prominent celebrities in 1969 based on the belief that they were evil and had murderous intentions toward members of the cult, and the members of the Branch Davidian cult directed by David Koresh and their violent confrontation with authority in Waco, Texas, in 1993. The leader foments the followers to enact his unintegrated rage toward others who are misperceived to be the bearers of the malignant intentions. The Westboro

Baptist Church in Topeka, Kansas, under the leadership of Fred Phelps, is a more recent example. It is organized around enactment of hatred toward homosexuals, veterans, and others who have been victims of catastrophes; based on religiously framed beliefs by Phelps and his wife that members of these groups have violated God's laws. The catastrophes are seen as part of their just punishment, and using righteous quotations from Biblical scripture, the cult believes it has the responsibility to act as the righteous punitive hand of God. Cults are small because they appeal to the most deranged minds: the most psychotic among the population, who are unable to live within any ordinary social community.

Larger organizations based on shared primordial mentation can be found among national governments and major religions. Religions are comprised of shared belief systems or ideologies. Nations can be loosely grouped as democratic, autocratic, or fascist. However, recent social awareness in the United States has raised the possibility that democracy may be a fictional ideal, as the so-called democracy Americans have wanted to believe they enjoy seems to have been a theocracy based on white male supremacy and systematic othering of those who do not fit those categories.

The penchant for ideologically based violence that characterizes religious extremism – such as Inquisition, Crusades, and Jihad – is a kind of fascism. But although religions are organized around systematic attribution of hostile evil intentions to non-believers, the majority of humans capable of reflective thought also accept religious belief as a normal even essential aspect of life and social groupings, and except in more extreme instances persons outside the belief system are simply thought of as non-believers and any misattribution of hostile intentions to them tends to be more ritualistic than enactive.

The demarcation between autocracy or dictatorship and fascism is not clear-cut. In general, it has to do with the presence or absence of shared ideology. Ideological unity is a prominent feature of fascism and is based on the delusion that following the leader and his beliefs will provide the people with the superior lives they believe they deserve. Fascist leaders like Hitler gain power because their ideology of disenfranchisement appeals to a wider spectrum of people than does that of a cult, which tends to attract persons who are psychotic. Followers come to believe that actualizing the ideology by extermination of those who are believed to be different and to be the impediments will be the solution to their sense of deprivation and frustration. Part of the attraction is the license or social sanction to express uncontrolled and unpunished rage in the form of violence toward designated others.

Dictatorship involves undifferentiation of leader from follower that is based more on fear than on wishful entitlement. Rather than licensing personal expression of hostility, it requires subjugation of any drive toward autonomy by those subjugated. The ideological othering element, encouraging members to enact hate toward and suspiciousness of groups of people identified as "other," is less well developed. Dictatorships are more common in less developed countries, whose citizens have traditionally been anonymous mistreated cogs in a larger machine and who have not developed the refined sense of individual rights and entitlement characteristic of contemporary western societies.

Of course, not all those who allow themselves to be subjugated by dictators and fascist leaders are psychotic. People who are not sufficiently secure to risk autonomous difference with powerful leaders are susceptible to the influence of leaders who not only threaten autonomous expression of difference but give permission for and reward regressive expression of fear and rage.

The results of the presidential elections, first of Donald Trump and then of Joseph Biden, have left many educated observers shocked to discover the large proportion of the population who support Trump and echo and promulgate his fascistic, illogical, unrealistic beliefs, and puzzled about the reasons why. Half a population cannot be psychotic as these conditions are basically social judgments of deviance. To understand this tsunami of support, it is first necessary to understand the various social groups that share primordial mental activity and then to understand the special circumstances in which their interests align so that they act synergistically.

One such group consists of persons who have been unable to form a stable attachment to a primary caregiver and develop a separate sense of self. These are the individuals who fit the description of psychosis in the previous chapters. They are particularly susceptible to involvement in movements that offer them a home for their beliefs and that license as acceptable actions that in another context would not only be unacceptable, but perhaps criminal.

Another group is comprised of members of orthodox social enclaves based on a particular kind of caring that is restricted to others who share a common belief system that is xenophobic and views anyone with a different opinion or way of thinking as enemy and dangerous. The 1960 movie *Inherit the Wind*, based on the so-called 1926 Scopes "monkey trial" in Dayton, Tennessee, is an iconic depiction of such a subculture organized around primordial mentation. It was galvanized into destructive action by external forces. The ACLU, then in its infancy, decided to challenge the anti-scientific, pro-religious Tennessee law prohibiting teaching of evolution in the schools. They led members of the Dayton community to believe they could gain national recognition of their beliefs by serving as a test case, and enlisted John T. Scopes, a substitute teacher who was not sure he had ever actually taught the theory of evolution, to challenge the law. They hired the well-known attorney Clarence Darrow and enlisted William Jennings Bryan, a deeply religious man who repudiated science, to represent the community. The result was the conversion of an otherwise more or less satisfied peaceful community into an inflamed destructive mob, aroused to hatred and violence.

Representative Marjorie Taylor Greene, who was chosen to represent a Republican enclave in rural Georgia near Appalachia during the Biden election, is a more recent example. Members of the tightly knit community she came to represent are xenophobic, but as they all agree with one another, they had no need to enact their hatred. When they elected Greene as their representative, however, her beliefs espoused expression of hatred of Muslims, Jews, Black people, anyone different from herself. She embraced conspiracy theories, including the belief that wealthy Jews using lasers from outer space were responsible for California wildfires, and she denied that events like the 9/11 destruction of the twin towers and some of the massive school shootings actually occurred. When interviewed subsequent to her congressional behavior, some members of the rural, farming community that elected her expressed surprise and embarrassment about the extreme expression of her views, but continued to support her basic positions, because the shared beliefs underlying them had unified their community for decades.

Other persons in the destructive coalition that supports Trump have been able to develop some sense of separate self and reflective thought but retain islands of primordial mental activity because of fundamental insecurity. These people are vulnerable to regression and are susceptible to the kind of "home" that shared belief systems and the temptation to license their expression of violence might offer. Many of the Republicans in the House who privately express reservations about Trump but publicly stand behind him out of fear of retaliation or loss of their positions of power seem to belong to this group.

Finally, some persons who operate from reflective thought but have acquired little or no sense of morals and ethics might exploit the extremism of these others for their own political purposes. The majority leader of the Senate Mitch McConnell and the leader of the House of Representatives Kevin McCarthy may fit this latter politicly opportunistic category.

The catalyst for this coalition and conflagration appears to have been the charismatic leadership of Donald Trump, whose socially successful employment of primordial mental functioning was described in Chapter 15 and appears to have been the result of extreme trauma and insecurity in the infantile stage of attachment and separation, leading to the need to control others and gain their unequivocal support. He provided the match that lit the incendiary explosive coalition of destructive forces; the coming together of psychotic persons, of large social groups organized around primordial mental activity, of persons susceptible to regression when offered a primordial belief "home," and opportunists who operated from reflective thought but exploited the growing movement for their own power-seeking purposes.

This eruption of human destructiveness is but the latest episode of a clash that has occurred repeatedly since social organizations first emerged in the Middle Ages based on individual self-actualization rather than the traditional ones in which persons were nothing more than cogs in a larger social entity. The subsequent iterations of this clash have pitted bastions of education and science, humanistic social organizations, and those who attempt to form governments based on reflective thought and respectful awareness of individual differences and rights against organizations based on the fundamental premise that only a single point of view and its advocates can exist. In its most recent American political incarnation, it has led to ongoing debate about whether this difference can be addressed and resolved "across the aisle," as the political saying goes, by the representatives of each point of view somehow understanding one another and agreeing that the difference is not one of mind and social organization, but of positions about important economic and social issues. A deeper understanding of the dual nature of human mind and the variety and immiscibility of social systems based on it suggests otherwise. I think it safe to say that the core of the chasm relates to the fact that the factions represent qualitatively different, immiscible ways that minds work. One supports the principle of awareness and respect for individual difference, self-control, and reflective efforts to determine what is real and true, whereas the other is based on fixed belief and conformity. The first involves curiosity and a search for truth and reality, the second begins with the conviction that wisdom has been received and rules must be complied with. The first is based on caring for others, whether or not they think as we do so long as they do not do tangible harm, whereas the second is xenophobic and views difference and disagreement as inherently dangerous and evil.

For this reason, communication between representatives of the two forms of mental activity is most likely impossible. The inevitable result is struggle for dominance, in which representatives of primordial mentation attempt to subdue, convert, or exterminate those who disagree, whereas representatives of reflective thought try to educate, and when that fails, fight to contain and control those who believe otherwise.

In the bigger picture, a compassionate reflective society must search for ways to identify and remediate the problems of human attachment and separation that lead to maladaptive destructive perpetuation of primordial mental activity and the social systems that arise from it. Perhaps the ultimate irony, however, is that the very focus on respect for individuality and caring based upon it that seems so necessary if civilization is to survive is also responsible for some of the destructiveness, especially related to unchecked expansion of the population, which threatens our species with extinction. This complexity is explored in the concluding chapters.

The next chapter is devoted to a broader consideration of the social organizations we group under the rubric of civilization. Civilization is comprised of a confusing interweaving of elements that are destructive and ones that are not. The distinction between the two is not always obvious. Some developments related to the emphasis of contemporary culture on individual or self-actualization that seems constructive appear very different if viewed from the perspective of the species as a whole.

17

CIVILIZATION AND THE CONFUSING INTERACTION OF CONSTRUCTIVE AND DESTRUCTIVE FORCES

If a group of thoughtful people were asked to choose a single word to describe the difference between humans and other species, let us say chimps as they are generally thought of as the animals that most closely resemble us, I suspect the terms most frequently chosen would be civilization and culture. Chapter 12 describes the evolution of human civilization from its presumptive primate group origins, fancifully depicted in the opening scene of Stanley Kubrick's 1967 movie *2001*. A chimp discovers it can use an animal bone as a weapon against a marauding enemy tribe, and after gleefully bludgeoning his opponent in combat, exultantly hurls it into the air, where it morphs into a spaceship in conquest of the universe, to the accompanying strains of Strauss's beautiful Blue Danube Waltz. If this same group were asked to choose adjectives and adverbs to evaluate civilization, I suspect most would choose such words as progressive, better, improvement, enlightenment, and achievement. Unfortunately, matters are not so simple. The notion of a super-social superiority species advanced by E. O. Wilson and shared by many others is markedly in contrast to much of the information reviewed in the preceding chapters. Although chimps are one of the few species that are purposely destructive to their fellows, the circumstances are circumscribed and very different than the destruction practiced by humans against one another; it usually involves bands of males encountering one another by accident and fighting hand and tooth over territory. While they apparently use simple weapons to kill prey for food, I know of no evidence that they are sufficiently "sophisticated" to use them against one another. A more realistic evolutionary movie scenario involving chimps and humans might have depicted a chimp hunting for food with a simple club that morphs into a nuclear weapon of mass destruction or a pill such as fentanyl responsible for so many addiction deaths. Perhaps a

DOI: 10.4324/9781003442318-17

more appropriate musical background would have been Berlioz's Symphonie Fantastique. But such a film would have had little box office appeal.

This chapter is about civilization, but not exactly in the usual sense, as it is a complex human achievement that cannot readily be pigeonholed into positive and negative categories, but does have some significant destructive aspects that set us apart from other species. The positive achievements of civilization and culture are well known. Many have written about Shakespeare and Bach far more eloquently than I could possibly do. I could also write about the multitude of ways that civilization in the form of science and technology has bettered the lot of many individual human beings, and doing so would be but one side of the coin. Instead, the chapter will explore the darker side of the self-centric culture that has evolved around the individual self: enhancement and amplification of the power of individual destructiveness toward the self, the social order, and our species. Science, technology, medicine, and public health are responsible for new forms of social destructiveness that are not always obvious. The enhancement of individual and social life that has been so positive is also responsible for such things as the gradual destruction of the natural environment, and a dramatic explosion in earth's population that threatens the survival of our and other species and the sufficiency of earth's resources to continue to sustain life itself. This chapter concentrates on the complexity of "progress" and the dark side of civilization and undertakes the difficult task of trying to separate constructive from destructive. Some of the complexity relates to the fact that such a determination depends upon context. Some of our most remarkable civilized achievements might be viewed as constructive or destructive, depending on the individual and social purposes for which they are used and the perspective from which they are viewed. What is considered constructive from the perspective of individual human beings might be destructive if viewed from the perspective of human society or the human species as a whole, and what might seem constructive from an immediate social perspective might be destructive in relation to alteration of the population and environment.

Domestication of species, especially animals, is a good example of this complexity. Its origins can be traced back thousands of years, literally to the dawn of civilized homo sapiens perhaps 12,000 years ago, and the shift from a hunter-gatherer to an agricultural culture. The domestication of other species has provided humans with many of what we consider the comforts of civilization – companionship, a readily available and controllable source of food, clothing, and other products in hitherto unimaginable variety that can be accumulated, stored, processed, and transported. No wonder that it coincided with the beginnings of civilized communities and population expansion both in size and in geographical scope, as Jared Diamond observed in his book *Guns, Germs and Steel* (1997). Diamond also points out that proximity to domestic species also introduced new diseases to humans. Domestication defined people's lives, producing shepherds and their flocks in the Middle East, Asia, and Europe and cowboys in the New World. These led to new forms of conflicts among groups; the cattlemen and the sheepmen; and the song "Don't Fence Me In." David Nibert (2013) calls the process "domesecration" because of its association with power and control, particularly with the destruction of other species and of the natural environment. I would add destruction of humans as well.

The association of civilization with destruction is vividly illustrated by examining the advent and effects of science and technology. These more recent civilized "advances" have produced large-scale means of social destruction. The creation of weapons that enhance the destructive scope and power of individual human beings is the example that most readily comes to mind. In 250 years, human tools of aggression have gone from the primitive ball and gunpowder cannons and muskets of the Revolution and the difficult to use single-shot rifles of the American Civil War that did not easily kill even a single human to guns and scopes to aim them precisely that even infants can and do inadvertently use them to kill people, and even worse, to nuclear weapons and intercontinental supersonic missiles that can decimate millions in a blinding flash by the simple press of a button. While the destructive potential of technology increases, the maturity of the people who have access to their products, particularly the world leaders who are empowered to make decisions about their use, does not. The United States and Russia are said to have a combined arsenal of 14,700 nuclear weapons and it is estimated that there are 15,700 nuclear weapons in existence worldwide. The potential destruction of human life and natural resources, and alteration of the climate and the earth's atmosphere that can ensue if an immature hostile individual like the former president of the United States whose impulse-ridden personality structure was elucidated in Chapter 15 or the current Russian Premier Vladimir Putin presses the button is unimaginable. In 1982, Brian Martin estimated that a US–Soviet nuclear exchange might kill 400–450 million directly, mostly in the United States, Europe, and Russia, and perhaps several hundred million more through delayed radiation effects. In 2008, a survey by the Future of Humanity Institute estimated a 4 percent probability of human extinction from warfare by 2100. However horrendous it is to look at this possibility from the perspective of valuation of human life, a case can be made from the perspective of the function of R in Wilson's formulation of social population regulation mechanisms that such mass destruction might serve to prune the population to levels the planet can sustain. More about this in the pages to come.

The potential of some of the technological "advances" that might inadvertently or through deliberate misuse cause mass destruction is equally complex. For example, our collective thirst for sources of energy and our use of chemical and mechanical means to extract the last ounce of resources from the environment may be enhancing some individual lives, but it is depleting and destroying the environment and poisoning countless others. An October 2017 report published in the *Lancet* stated that toxic air, water, and soil were collectively responsible for nine million deaths worldwide in 2015, particularly from air pollution which was linked to deaths by increasing susceptibility to noninfectious diseases, such as heart disease, stroke, and lung cancer.

Nick Bostrom's book *Superintelligence: Paths, Dangers, Strategies* details still less obvious destructive risks posed by artificial intelligence (AI). At this writing, there is serious discussion about whether AI can replicate everything that is essentially human, including creativity and emotion, so successfully that robots can not only fool humans but perhaps replace them. Recently, AI programs have been developed that produce manuscripts so impressive that it is difficult to determine whether or not they are produced by humans, and chat programs and search engines with responses so convincing that they have been very upsetting and destructive to human participants. Meanwhile, more and more technologically manufactured parts are being transplanted into humans, even the human brain, also blurring the distinction between human and machine. Science can now alter DNA, and nanotechnology has the potential to create increasingly autonomous self-replicating robots that might someday be used to gain destructive power over human life and resources. Stephen Hawking predicted that AI could "spell the end of the human race."

Recently, a new kind of creature was announced: living robots. Researchers from the University of Vermont and Tufts University created these tiny creatures from frog stem cells using a supercomputer to design the arrangement of cells. Named after the frog species from which the stem cells came (*Xenopus laevis*, the African clawed frog) and containing between 500 and 1,000 cells, these living things (they are frogs yet not frogs) can move, self-organize, and carry tiny pellets in their center when designed in a donut shape. They have the potential to carry medication to specific areas of the body, scrape plaque from arteries, and clear toxic waste. No word yet on their classification among other living things, though some of them have little protuberances on the bottom, possibly making them into "quadrupeds." Presumably, they might have more malignant potential uses as well.

Biotechnology can now genetically alter viruses, plant, animal, and human life in ways that are directly intended to be harmful to human life or might indirectly have consequences beyond those for which they were intended. In 2008, a survey by the Future of Humanity Institute estimated a 2 percent probability of extinction from engineered pandemics by 2100. Some still believe that the COVID-19 virus was engineered in a Wuhan laboratory in the course of biological weapon research and inadvertently escaped its boundaries, as in Stephen King's fascinating novel *The Stand,* whose plot was summarized in Chapter 3.

Among the myriad of forces of human destructiveness wrought by civilization, perhaps the least appreciated and discussed is the current rate of growth of the human population and its causes and potential consequences. This is a result of social evolution from holistic sociocentric groupings prior to the industrial revolution in which individual members functioned as selfless cogs to a society that increasingly values and seeks to enhance each individual life, often heedless of the consequences to the larger group and the species.

Chapter 12 traced the evolution of culture and society from its earliest "uncivilized" social groupings through social-centric cultures based on shared primordial mentation to the so-called age of reason and enlightenment and the industrial revolution that accompanied it, which brought with it an awakening of the concept of individuality. An important dimension of this evolution has been the decentering from sociocentric life organized around the local fiefdom (the Lord of the Manor) and the Church (also around the Lord, but this time "king of kings and lord of lords"), under whose joint jurisdiction humans were interchangeable parts whose individual destinies were of no consequence and whose function was to sustain the system. The result was reconstitution of the world into new forms of social organization based on science, technology, and industry, which valued individual creativity as well as the will of the Lords. Consider the fact that the telephone, the radio, the automobile and the airplane, antibiotics, drugs to control heart failure and cancer, body part replacement surgeries, and more were all virtually unknown only a century ago, to say nothing of vast improvements in public health and sanitation.

Another change was the advent of colonialism around the time of the industrial revolution; the drive of social groups to multiply in numbers, assets and power, expand their territories, and expropriate and exploit captive lands and peoples. The missionary zeal of self-centric cultures was initially driven by religion and the conviction that those of the faith were bringing civilization to the savages and the heathen. It was further fueled by the desire of individuals to acquire more power and resources, by the development of technologies that facilitate destruction of enemies, and ultimately by the corporate desire to expand. Colonialism is associated with religion and monarchy, but we joke that wherever we go in the world there will be a McDonald's. Tribal and spiritual cultures that do not possess either the technology or the urge to expand cannot compete with self-centric cultures because their implicit goal is equilibrium, so they have gradually been overrun and taken over.

In the expanding world of self-centric cultures, individual lives that would ordinarily have been aborted to begin with, or severely foreshortened by genetic abnormality, disease, aging, and natural disaster, are now not only humanely preserved because of the belief each one of us is a uniquely valuable human being, but consistent with the ideal of self-actualization, given educational opportunities for personal growth and accomplishment that were unimaginable, for example, in the sociocentric culture of the Middle Ages. As traditional sociocentric cultures and subcultures have been gradually colonized by and assimilated into self-centric thinking, members who accepted without reflection the status of anonymous cogs in a larger social unity inexorably acquire a new perspective that they have been poorly treated as individual selves. They have increasingly adopted the self-centric belief that they are entitled to lives of consequence; to "life, liberty and the pursuit of happiness."

In the course of the gradually changing organization of society, the preservation, enhancement, and actualization of each individual life has gradually become more important than the welfare, viability, and fate of the social group as a whole. One effect of medicine and public health has been to attenuate the impact of disease that in times past would have culled the population. For example, epidemics and pandemics that regularly decimated a large percentage of population, such as the bubonic plague in the fourteenth century that is believed to have eliminated 60 percent of the population of Europe, have been mitigated if not eradicated. Discovery of the role of pathogens in disease and related developments in sanitation and public health as well as the invention of antibiotics and vaccines have enabled vast numbers of people to survive who would otherwise have died. Diseases like smallpox, polio, HIV, swine flu, SARS, and Ebola, any of which might have led to a pandemic in the past and decimated a large proportion of the human race, have been limited and contained.

The cardiologist Eric Topol wrote an op-ed piece in the March 2019 *New York Times* that illustrates some of the ramifications of the culture of the self. He wrote:

> I participated in a two-week experiment that involved using a smartphone app to track every morsel of food I ate, every beverage I drank and every medication I took, as well as how much I slept and exercised. I wore a sensor that monitored my blood-glucose levels, and I sent in a sample of my stool for an assessment of my gut microbiome. All of my data, amassed with similar input from more than a thousand other people, was analyzed by artificial intelligence to create a personalized diet algorithm. The point was to find out what kind of food I should be eating to live a longer and healthier life.

On the surface of it, none of the resources that when into the intensive study of what was best for him seems to have been directly destructive, but what are the consequences for humankind of the implication that such an expenditure of resources on a single life is not only a justified but a desirable goal?

The technologies that function to save, enhance, and prolong human lives that would otherwise not have come into being to begin with, or would have been ended by defects, diseases, and simple aging, have a dark side from the perspective of population growth and conservation of resources. Not so long-ago humans did not name children until well along in childhood as so many did not survive, and the average life span was three decades. Infant mortality has been drastically curtailed even among those with significant birth defects, and life span has nearly tripled. The preservation and enhancement of individual life through advances in medicine, public health, and education has generated an unprecedented growth of the population. As long ago as 1798, Thomas Malthus observed that as the average person's nutrition improves the population grows, and while the food supply increases arithmetically, the population grows exponentially. Since then, earth has supported an explosive exponential growth in population and gradual destruction of other species and the natural environment that is essential to maintain it, leading to scarcity of habitable space and life-sustaining resources, and as a result, the looming threat of extinction of the entire human species to say nothing of other plant and animal life.

It has been estimated that over the first 200,000 or so years of human existence prior to the industrial revolution, during which period cultures were sociocentric and self-sustaining but not expansive in nature, the world population grew very slowly, eventually reaching one billion around 1700. The population grew by 600 million in the two centuries prior to 1900. In another half century, by 1950, almost one billion were added and the population reached 2.5 billion. Now, less than 75 years later, it is an estimated eight billion; a remarkable eightfold explosion in the past three centuries. This despite the appalling toll on human life of such things as two world wars, several epidemics and two pandemics, and multiple instances of genocide.

Taking into account evidence that the overall birth rate is declining, it is estimated that the population will rise to 8.6 billion by 2030, 9.8 billion by 2050, and an unimaginable 11.2 billion by the turn of the next century, a potential catastrophe for the species and the planet that does not get nearly so much attention, for example, as how much the sea level is projected to rise in a comparable time span. Habitable space is becoming increasingly scarce as are life-sustaining resources. David Pimentel, professor of ecology and agriculture at Cornell University, and Mario Giampietro, senior researcher at the National Research Institute on Food and Nutrition (INRAN), in their 1994 study *Food, Land, Population and the U.S. Economy*, estimate that the maximum population that the United States can sustain is about 200 million. They concluded that the United States must reduce its population by at least one-third, and that world population would need to be reduced by two-thirds if our species is to survive.

The ascending population trajectory has not been without bumps in the road, however. Humans have played an increasing role in creating and perpetuating communicable diseases that decimate the population. The recent COVID-19 pandemic is an example. Even if the virus itself was not created in a laboratory and inadvertently spread, as some believe, humans appear to have played a part in its jumping species from bats. The Wuhan market in China is a crowded place in a densely populated city that sells a mélange of inadequately refrigerated bird, fish, and animal products under less than sanitary condition. And the ease and frequency of world travel have contributed to a wildfire spread of disease that might in the days of yore been more readily contained.

Medical technology and the increasing focus on women's right to lives not fettered by enforced uncontrolled breeding have also combined to lead to an increasing focus on birth control and raised the possibility that it might halt or even reverse the population explosion. As women become better educated and more aware of their rights as individuals to control their destinies and the quality of their lives, the birth rate in so-called developed parts of the world, particularly Europe, the UK, and Japan, has declined and no longer outstrips the death rate. Women are bearing fewer children, and many are choosing not to become mothers at all. A handful of studies of male fertility conducted in major cities in the United States and Europe over the past 50 years suggest that it is progressively declining as well for reasons that no one seems to understand. The population balance is shifting toward dominance by older people beyond childbearing age.

The use of birth control might become more widespread if a concerted effort is made to encourage the emancipation and education of African women, as Africa is projected to experience by far the largest population growth in the coming century. The conflict inherent in such an idea is that these same emancipated women who might decide to limit their pregnancies will expect better lives for themselves that require them to have a greater share of the earth's scarce resources. And once again, in a curious way, technology is rising to the challenge, providing new and sophisticated techniques that enable infertile couples to bear children and freezing of eggs so that female childbearing years are extended. The estimates of continuing explosive expansion of the population over the coming century, however, do take into account a progressive decline in the birth rate from 2.5 births per woman currently to a projected 2.0 by 2100.

In summary, the dual nature of mind that distinguishes humans from other animals and that results from the lengthy period of immaturity and learning subsequent to birth has enabled civilization's monumental achievements. Ironically, our advanced civilization is also responsible for the devastating destructiveness that seems to differentiate humans from other animals and threaten the survival of our species and of the planet on which it depends.

Even more confusing is the fact that our civilized achievements have improved the survival, duration, and quality of individual lives, but that very fact has led to an explosive expansion of population that threatens the earth's resources. It is difficult to untangle the effect of the destructive forces that appear to be expanding the human population in unprecedented ways from those reducing it. What will be the ultimate balance between pruning of the population to a level consistent with species survival, whether unintentionally in acts of overt destruction or ones more deliberate and potentially constructive, and the forces, intentional or inadvertent that are leading to unchecked expansion of the population? At the moment, the scales seem heavily tipped toward a condition where the human species will overrun the earth and devastate its resources, a scenario far different than the success E. O. Wilson likened to that of ants, whose capacity for expansion he likened to humans. Woody Guthrie laments the sinking of the *Titanic* in his historic ballad. But its passengers were by and large an affluent, privileged group of individuals. If the great ship homo sapiens (or is it homo destrudo?) goes down, will it do so at the same time that we, the passengers, are enjoying individual lives of unprecedented meaning and prosperity beyond the wildest imaginations of "primitive" peoples?

18

IMPLICATIONS OF A PSYCHOANALYTIC UNDERSTANDING OF THE HUMAN DIFFERENCE BASED ON A REVISED THEORY OF EVOLUTION FOR SOCIETY AND FOR THE FATE OF OUR SPECIES

The development and eventual configuration of the human mind are both qualitatively different from that of other animal species. While this difference, like all others that separate species, is driven by biological evolution, biology alone cannot account for it. Much human development occurs subsequent to birth and involves learned acquisition of a process of reflective thought, which, in turn, enables complex learning from experience, and acquisition of knowledge that can be passed down and accumulated from one generation to the next. The psychoanalytic theory of development, especially the formation of the complex nature of the human mind through the vicissitudes of attachment, separation, and individuation, is uniquely valuable in understanding this process. The human difference calls into question the accepted belief that evolution is an exclusively biological process and privileges psychoanalysis and its companion social sciences sociology and cultural anthropology as ways to comprehend its uniqueness.

The question about the nature and origin of uniquely human destructiveness, in turn, opens the possibility for expanding the scope of psychoanalysis which was foreclosed by Freud. Freud erroneously assumed that basic biological processes that he called instincts function as mental motivations that he called drives, without explaining how this leap from instincts to mental drives occurs. And he also failed to recognize and account for the human difference when he assumed destructiveness is similarly motivated and understood in all species. I believe he confused the basic biological processes underlying life and death in all species other than humans with needs for maintenance of homeostasis that Hans Selye (1946) identified. The basic biological processes responsible for fertilization and germination, birth, growth, decay, and death do not require mental representation and awareness. These are the existential

DOI: 10.4324/9781003442318-18

givens of all life forms. In order to maintain living homeostasis, humans and other animals are aware of needs related to hunger, thirst, evacuation, temperature regulation, and procreation. Awareness of distinctive urges to destroy has other origins and other meanings in humans. When well cared for infants cry or complain, it is because they are aware of needs: hungry, thirsty, or in physical discomfort, without yet having the sophisticated knowledge to be able to understand and articulate what they are. Otherwise, they are cheerful and curious to learn, not driven to destroy themselves. In any case, Freud failed to account for two essential matters. The first is the human difference: the nature, extent, and virulence of destructiveness in homo sapiens compared to other species. The second is the process by which biological instinct becomes psychic representation and motivation. He further directed attention away from the need for psychoanalysis to understand more about the problem of human destructiveness by focusing his theoretical and clinical attention on the life force, the libidinal drive and its developmental vicissitudes. His idiosyncratic focus has for the most part been passed on to subsequent generations of analysts, so that psychoanalysis has not grappled directly with the unique nature, origins, and significance of human destructiveness. Consideration of the so-called death instinct has been relegated to something of a speculative philosophical exercise that is optional but not foundational for further elaboration of the theory of mind.

It is not the case that the study of human destructiveness has failed to focus on psychology, sociology, and cultural anthropology, however. The very discipline of psychoanalysis is founded on understanding human destructiveness. But by not linking these human problems to their uniquely human origins, by failing to provide a satisfactory account of the leap from body and biology to mind and behavior, Freud did not open the door to linking a psychoanalysis of mind and behavior to the basic biology of species, and therefore linking it to neuroscience in the way he had hoped and making it as imperative to study as biology. A theory that harkens back to biology but focuses on understanding the transformation to psychological motivation, and that emphasizes the difference between humans and other species, makes understanding human destructiveness one of the central problems in psychoanalysis, potentially enlarges the theory of evolution, and places psychoanalysis in a position to make a fundamental contribution to society now and to the problem of the future of our species.

Much contemporary social dialogue has been spent discussing the crucially important question of what, if anything, we humans are able and willing to do to mitigate and prevent our remarkable destructiveness and to preserve a viable social structure now and for immediate future generations. Understanding what is unique about the human mind and its causal evolutionary role places psychoanalysis in the forefront of possible ameliorating intervention. Neoteny has required us to learn in a way that distinguishes humans from other species. But it has complicated the learning process with the problems that may arise during the phase of attachment, separation, and development of thinking in such a way as to promote destructive as well as constructive consequences. Difficult as it is, society needs to consider ways of dealing with the rights and responsibilities of bearing children in such a way as to make it more likely that infants will have an opportunity to grow with the help of loving parents. And we need to develop ways of detection and early intervention in instances where the process of attachment and separation is going awry. A tall order, indeed!

The predominant social concern about destruction needs to shift from urgent but symptomatic manifestations of environmental and species destruction and their amelioration to broader considerations of root causes. With those in mind, society needs to face the urgent issues related to what, if anything, we are willing to do to address these root causes, in light of the fact that what is necessary may run counter to some of our basic values and assumptions.

It seems fitting that the major focus of this final chapter, which brings us to the conclusion of the book on human destructiveness, is on human finality, the relationship of human destructiveness to the survival and extinction of our species. This question proves to be particularly complex, as many aspects of our civilization and the focus on individual rights, entitlement, gratification, welfare, and social values have a darker side that threatens the human species with a very early extinction because we privilege individual life over social and species survival, and in so doing, ensure that the explosive expansion of population that is destroying other life and earth's resources, and hence ourselves, will continue. Do we humans care enough about survival to make hard choices that challenge some of our most cherished individual and social beliefs, values, and rights?

The average life span of a species is 5–10 million years, though invertebrate species have a span about ten times that of vertebrates. It is estimated that homo sapiens is about 200,000 years old (May, Lawton & Stork, 1995). In other words, homo sapiens is a newborn amongst species, and yet there is already substantial reason to be concerned about our extinction.

Most scenarios optimists tend to envision for saving humankind and our planet and making our world ever better can be classified in three categories that are not necessarily mutually exclusive: technological fantasies, eusociality beliefs, and religious mythologies.

In techno-fantasy, when earth's resources are exhausted or hopelessly contaminated and the planet becomes arid and toxic, advances in technology will make it possible to sustain civilization in ways now unimaginable, or else the remaining humans will migrate to another planet (and who knows what will happen there?). Those with enthusiasm for such beliefs, including not only novelists and film makers in search of plots that will sell but persons like Elon Musk, may well overestimate human ingenuity and good will and underestimate the formidable nature of the problems attendant both to human destructiveness and imagined techno-salvation. And they may overlook that technology has not only done little to ameliorate the problems so far, but it has also probably done more to worsen them. Technology has enabled newer and more powerful forms of destruction. It taxes credulity to believe the leaders of the world's powers are likely to agree to curtail the use of technologies to exploit the environment on which we depend sufficiently to preserve it, or voluntarily and unilaterally stop manufacturing weapons of mass destruction and destroy stockpiles of weapons, given the paranoid mistrust nations have of one another.

On the other hand, it is possible that the blatant human penchant for destructiveness represents what Wilson in his earlier theory referred to as R, destructiveness that serves to prune a population to sustainable levels. If so, it has failed, as the advent of technology that has caused the problem is paralleled by an astonishing expansion of the population. Technology in the form of public health and medicine has enabled the preservation and enhancement of individual human life and in so doing contributed powerfully to unchecked population growth.

The human penchant for idealism generates eusociality fantasies about the supposedly extraordinary human capacity for social collaboration that ignore reality. The lion will lay down with the lamb so to speak, and through enlightened negotiation and cooperation, different nations, genders, ethnicities, races, religions, and other mutually hostile social groups will recognize their common cause, learn to respect one another, and live peaceably and constructively side by side, despite an ever more crowded world where people are propelled into competition for increasingly scarce resources. If history is any teacher, this belief is unlikely to move beyond the realm of wishful thinking. Most humans seem too self-interested, too acquisitive, too power-hungry, and too immersed in the current moment to foresee future consequences to themselves, to say nothing of future generations with sufficient vividness to be willing to tighten our collective belts, postpone gratification, use self-control, trust one another, respect one another's views, and make major sacrifices of the luxuries technology has afforded in anticipation of bringing about a world many of us will not get to experience ourselves. The particular irony of such beliefs is that the social organizations of other species, however deprived they may be of vocal apparatus and frontal lobe complexity, are organized around sociocentric rather than self-centric principles, so that the goal of the ultimate welfare of the group appears to be much more benign and collaborative than that of humans.

Mythology is another popular source of belief about the continuity of human life in the face of destructiveness, embodied most powerfully in contemporary religions. There are two general classes of religious myths.

Chapter 3 explains how they share a belief that humans are everlasting and that the species will never truly become extinct. One tells of endless repetition of a cycle of birth and death. Buddhist belief in successive reincarnations is an example. In the other, there is an end to the world as we know it, but not an end to everything human or humanoid. A few humans survive to repopulate the world, or else humankind is transformed to an exalted plane of being. Although we are skeptical of the truth value of such beliefs when we think of them in relation to ancient cultures such as those of Greece, Egypt, and pre-Columbian Mesoamerica and call them myths, the same reasoning is seldom applied to ideas large numbers of people in contemporary culture passionately cling to, perhaps as a kind of narcotic, to avoid facing a sense of urgency, helplessness, and foreboding related to more sobering reality about mortality and what science tells us about life and death. For that reason, far from helping save humankind, mythology actually encourages passivity and the belief that we will somehow live on regardless of what becomes of our mortal coil.

Many individuals and groups are making sincere efforts to bring about more national and international collaboration to reduce greenhouse gas emissions, save forests, preserve other species, and seek alternative forms of energy for the ever-increasing demands of humankind and to preserve endangered species. However much such efforts might mitigate the manifestations of destructiveness, they are symptomatic fixes. None of them address the root causes. Probably the greatest and least recognized threat to the human species is the eightfold explosion of population in the last three centuries, after being relatively stable for thousands of years, fueled by self-centric social organization, the industrial revolution, and the advent and proliferation of sophisticated technology. Even though there are some signs that population growth is slowing, the culture of the individual and the changes in social structure that have created it and their manifestations clearly indicate that the problems persist.

The larger problem is the human difference. That relates to evolution and how we understand it. Evolution of species is basically biological; there cannot be any argument about that. However, the currently accepted theory of evolution does not readily account for the mental and cultural developments that make humans unique. They do not fit neatly into the hypothesis that mutations produce phenotypes, and in turn, the phenotypes most favorable to species survival tend to survive. Many of the developments we think of as products of civilization do not appear to make our species more likely to survive, and the extent and virulence of human destructiveness certainly does not. However, the biological fact of neoteny that distinguishes humans from other species, enables and requires that humans learn from caregivers and develop a second mental structure, reflective thought. The complex knowledge that results cumulates and is transmitted from one generation to another and acts as a causal force, independent of biology. In other words, the theory of evolution needs to be modified to include the possibility that learned knowledge, transmitted from one generation to the next, can act as an evolutionary force independent of biology. What are the implications of this novel understanding of human evolution for the future of our species?

The first possibility is that far from being the superior species humans have wished to believe we are, whether from a religious or scientific vantage point, neoteny and the consequences arising from it, the prolonged extrauterine period of maturation and learning that distinguishes us from other animals, might be the consequence of a fatal flaw or mutation that will doom our species to an early exit from the world. Our extraordinary accomplishments in civilization and culture may contain the seeds of our destruction. While the jury is not in, evidence suggests that far from our smug belief that we humans represent the pinnacle of species evolution, our unique capacity for reflective thought that we prize so much may be a fatal defect resulting from a genetic mutation. It is easier to imagine an asteroid striking earth and destroying all life or even another Krakatoa magnitude volcanic eruption blocking sunlight and filling the air with pollution for years so that all life dies than it is to accept such an idea.

A second possibility is based on the hypothesis that E. O. Wilson's first, unitary model of social structure that he believed applies to all species does apply to humans as well, contradicting his later life optimistic assumptions about the human species. In other words, we are not the eusocial super-collaborative resourceful species he imagined in his later writings and supported by likening humans to ants, a flawed comparison that I explained in an earlier chapter. We would need to accept that despite the disparity between the virulent and seemingly purposeless nature of human destruction, it serves the same purpose, maintenance of a homeostatic balance between species size and available resources that individual destruction serves in sociocentric species. Were that the case, we would have to embrace every possibility for culling the population, no matter how horrifying and reprehensible and unacceptable they may seem from an individual or self-centric perspective.

The third possibility is complex in a different way but leads to some of the same practical considerations and decisions. It is that the unusual capacity for civilized reflective thinking and learning that distinguishes humans might also have gifted us with an unusual capacity to grasp, control, and reverse our equally unusual capacity for individual, social, and species destructiveness sufficiently to turn the ship around, as it were, before it hits the iceberg of extinction and sinks.

If the most likely possibility, that what makes humans unique is the phenotypic manifestation of a fatal mutation that will doom our species to extinction, is correct, then there is nothing we can do. In the closing pages, let us explore what humans can do proceeding from one of the other hypotheses, that our species conforms to the same principles that govern other species or that it does not, but that the creativity that distinguishes us might open vistas that can turn the tide of human destructiveness in a direction that might save our species, though at a cost that most of us might consider too expensive for our psychological pocketbooks.

When we think of saving humankind and preserving our planet, most of us think of curtailing the destruction of our environment and of other species and limiting development and use of technologies that enable human destruction on a hitherto unimaginable scale. Laudable as such beliefs are, they are at best symptomatic fixes that do not address root causes.

The two remaining hypotheses, though different from one another, lead to similar conclusions and problems, if for the moment one considers that the goal is survival of the human species, whatever the cost. Wilson's unitary model assumes that the species-centric purpose of destructiveness that he called R is to reduce the size of a population to a stable manageable equilibrium with available resources. The unchecked expansion of humankind is increasingly overburdening the earth and endangering its natural and animate resources. Can the unique human creativity that has produced the remarkable achievements of culture and civilization devise solutions to the problems created by human destructiveness?

While nations and their leaders seem to think nothing of the consequences for individual human beings of using the latest technologies to invent and stockpile weapons of mass destruction and of sending off armies of human youth to fight one another to the death, it is ironic that it is next to unthinkable that in the individual-centric culture and era in which we live, we would agree to let our fellow humans die and risk death ourselves from medically remediable conditions or horrible diseases when scientific knowledge related to personal and public health and advanced technologies exist to prevent such things. No reflective thoughtful human being will voluntarily choose to let nature take its course when loved ones face life or death situations, even though the result of enlightened intervention may be further increases in the population, consumption, and destruction of scarce resources and the likelihood of still more plagues in the future.

One method of reducing the population that most ostensibly enlightened people agree upon is birth control. However, China tried limiting family size but abandoned the policy, and it seems unlikely that the world powers, competing for dominance, would voluntarily agree to reduce the size of their populations or that governments would have the means to enforce such legislation. Most religions, Catholicism being the most blatant example, have value systems that reward large families and condemn those who choose not to reproduce. The use of birth control might become more widespread if a concerted effort is made to encourage the emancipation and education of African women, as Africa is projected to experience by far the largest population growth in the coming century. The conflict inherent in such an idea is that these same emancipated women who might decide to limit their pregnancies will expect better lives for themselves that require them to have a greater share of earth's scarce resources. And once again, in a curious way, technology is rising to the challenge, providing new and sophisticated techniques that enable infertile couples to bear children and freezing of eggs so that female child-bearing years are extended.

The concept of individual human life being expendable in the service of the goal of reducing population to a sustainable level, which might involve turning our backs to those who suffer and are in danger and allowing nature to take its course, is deeply repugnant to humans who have acquired the capacity for reflective thought and moral reasoning. Tribal cultures, whose social organization is based on primordial mentation, do not appear to have this problem. Members of the Piraha tribal culture described in Chapter 11 are able to do this while continuing to care about one another as their shared primordial mentation lacks a sense of the passage of time and the capacity to imagine consequences that for us seem intolerably painful. The husband of the woman suffering from protracted labor because the fetus was in a breech position until she eventually died was not overly troubled because he was unaware of what was going to happen. And after she died, when asked where his wife was, he answered "she is not here now." The parents allowing their infant to play with a sharp knife were not especially worried because they did not entertain the possibility of a future catastrophe. Perhaps, at least in this context, our capacity for reflective thought serves as a kind of curse that reminds us of unpleasant consequences to us as individuals if we take measures necessary to cull the population compatible with Wilson's concept of R.

One of the unpleasant consequences humans might need to think more deeply about involves confronting the contradictions that allow us to use technology, both to expand the population and to destroy it, without fundamental examination of the contradiction that might enable us to make an intelligent choice. Contemporary human beings, steeped in the social culture of self-actualization, use advances in science, medicine, and public health to enable and preserve individual life regardless of the social drain and population expansion that result from such things as supporting persons with genetic defect, the consequences of serious disease, horrendous accidents, and aged individuals who do not contribute to sustaining the social fabric. A result is the threefold increase in the average life span and an eightfold growth of the population in a little more than a century. Please do not put down the book and conclude I am a heartless monster. My personal choices and my understanding of the evolutionary trajectory of our species are different. Personally, my decisions are made based on valuation of individual human life. However, we need to consider the larger context, survival or extinction of our species, as well.

If we reach what seems an obvious conclusion from evidence presented that the human population needs to be drastically culled if our species is to survive and that among the myriad possibilities that this might happen, some scenarios are more constructive than others, then the question arises about whether there are more and less thoughtful ways this goal might be achieved. With this in mind, there are, in fact, precedents. Allocation of scarce resources is one. We seldom think of what happens to the person who is turned down at a university, or for a life-sustaining job, or in a state of desperation and destitution from application at the border to immigrate to this land of opportunity. Other examples of triage, choices to let some die and others live, date back at least to the Judeo-Christian Bible. The fabled Ark is an example of triage, setting limits that involved selection of representative couples of each species to board the vessel headed away from extinction. The Bible neglects to tell us what fate befell most of their fellows. Current examples of such triage all seem to involve situations of forced choice, such as the sinking of the *Titanic*, the triage that occurs in frontline first aid tents during war, and the decisions some hospitals overwhelmed with COVID-19 cases have had to make about who to treat and who must be turned away. Some science fiction novels and movies about the need to leave earth for another planet because life cannot be sustained here involve triage as well: the idea that not everyone can go. The problem with this, of course, is that the science involved is so far removed from any real immediate possibility that the issue of transporting billions of people to some other place in the universe or deciding who can and cannot go has yet to be taken seriously. It is human nature not to want to make such decisions unless forced by immediate unavoidable circumstances, but if we look beyond the immediate, the alternative of extinction might be considered a forced choice situation.

The previous discussion has been based upon the fact that the two mental processes, primordial mentation that humans share with members of other species and reflective representational thought that is unique to humans, have important bearing on whether and how we relate our current thinking and social structure to the long-term fate of the human species. The capacity of members of tribal cultures organized around primordial mentation to overlook the lethal or potentially lethal suffering of fellow members while still caring about them is a reflection of what E. O. Wilson called R, behavior designed to regulate the health of their social organization in relation to available resources and as a result, insure survival of the species. This is a two-sided coin, however, as tribal members are unable to envision a future; hence, the notion of species and survival is not in their cosmology. The Piraha built balsam models of the float plane that landed on the Maci River each time outside observers arrived but abandoned the pursuit after a very short time only to begin anew the next time such an event occurred. Reflective representational thought, on the other hand, has enabled us to consider such possibilities and even develop a biological science of evolution. Paradoxically, however, the capacity for thought has evolved as part of the evolution of self-centered social groupings, consisting of people who value immediate self-gratification and the maintenance and enhancement of their individual lives over significant belt-tightening activities and certainly over the outrageous idea of making deliberate decisions to withhold potential help and let fellow humans die, in the service of preserving the world for future generations and mitigating toward survival of the human species. That means we tend to bemoan consequences when it is too late to do anything about them. We tend to be a lock the barn door after the horse has escaped culture when dealing with major tragedies that could readily have been foreseen and forestalled by taking proactive measures.

Where does psychoanalysis fit in dealing with these large questions that confront humankind? The companion volume, *What Makes Humans Unique*, described the independent evolutionary force of the human mind that is capable of reflective representational thought that enables us to ask questions such as this book has posed, as well as to generate the kind of destructiveness that places our species in jeopardy. Psychoanalytic theory of attachment, separation, and early development inform us about how the human mind develops. Psychoanalysis, along with two other disciplines that originated around the same time, sociology and cultural anthropology, help us to think about these questions.

Psychoanalysis embraces both a theory of mind and a practical clinical application that is a child of the same self-centric human culture that has generated the population explosion that threatens the survival of our species. The clinical application is a therapy designed to preserve and enhance otherwise destructive individual human lives, and in so doing, indirectly enhance the social organizations in which these individuals play essential roles. In other words, psychoanalysis plays a paradoxical and in some respects contradictory role in regard to species survival, and in that respect is similar to many other contradictions I have described, especially in the areas of science and technology since the industrial revolution and the advent of reflective thought and the culture of the self. Speaking for a moment from the perspective of a psychoanalyst whose career has been devoted to trying to help the most severely disturbed destructive persons rather than from the perspective of species evolution and extinction of this chapter, the prospect of abandoning the use of psychoanalytic knowledge to help people seems anathema.

If I have left you, the reader, more thoughtful about the human difference, pointed out contradictions, and raised vexing questions about what in our nature is constructive and what destructive, then the book has achieved its purpose. Freud concluded his WWII correspondence with Einstein about the future of humanity pessimistically. I wish I could conclude with cheerful optimism, as have many of the mongers of human superiority and endless progress whose names and ideas have filled some of the pages of this book. My intent has not been to marvel about the superior nature of human beings, nor has it been to advocate behavior many of us find morally reprehensible. My goal has been to challenge prevalent conceptions about animal nature, the human difference, and the theory of evolution, and explore possible consequences of the choices we wittingly or unwittingly make. It is my hope that by facing this complexity rather than ignoring it, we might arrive at a position that is more consistent and realistically hopeful, if difficult, from which my offspring like those of you, the reader, will benefit.

REFERENCES

Ainsworth, M. (1982). Attachment: Retrospect and prospect. In C. Parkes & J. Stevenson-Hinde (Eds.) *The Place of Attachment in Human Behavior* (pp. 3–30). New York: Basic Books.

Ainsworth, M., Blehar, M., Waters, E., & Wall, S. (1978). *Patterns of Attachment: A Psychological Study of the Strange Situation*. Hillsdale, NJ: Erlbaum.

American Psychiatric Association (1952 1974). *Diagnostic and Statistical Manual*. New York: American Psychiatric Association Press.

Atwood, M. (2003). *Oryx & Crake*. London: Bloomsbury Press.

Bayeh, T., Tuomi, T., Almgren, P., et al. (2016). DNA methylation of loci within ABCG1 and PHOSPHO1 in blood DNA is associated with future type 2 diabetes risk. *Epigenetics*, 7: 482–488.

Bednarik, R. (2011). *The Human Condition*. New York: Springer.

Bell, D. (2022). Psychoanalytic reflections on the conditions of possibility of human destructiveness. *International Journal of Psycho-Analysis*, 103: 674–691.

Bergmann, M. (1992). *In the Shadow of Moloch: The Sacrifice of Children and Its Impact on Western Religions*. New York: Columbia University Press.

Bickerton, D. (1990). *Language and Species*. Chicago, IL: University of Chicago Press.

Bion, W. (1951). *Experiences in Groups*. New York: Basic Books.

Blair, G. (2015). *The Trumps: Three Generations of Builders and a Presidential Candidate*. New York: Simon & Schuster.

Bleuler, E. (1911a). *Textbook of Psychiatry*. New York: MacMillan (1924).

Bleuler, E. (1911b). *Dementia Praecox or the Group of Schizophrenias*. New York: International Universities Press (1950).

Boas, F. (1911). *The Mind of Primitive Man*. New York: The MacMillan Company (1938); London: Andesite Press (2017).

Bogin, B. (1997). Evolutionary hypotheses for human childhood (PDF). *Yearbook of Physical Anthropology*, 40: 63–89.

Boston Change Process Study Group (BCPSG) (2007). The foundational level of psychodynamic meaning: Implicit process in relation to conflict, defense and the dynamic unconscious. *International Journal of Psychoanalysis*, 88: 843–860.

Bostrom, N. (2014). *Superintelligence: Paths, Dangers, Strategies*. London: Oxford University Press.

Bowlby, J. (1969). *Attachment and Loss, Vol. I: Attachment*. London: Hogarth Press and the Institute of Psycho-Analysis.

Bowlby, J. (1973). *Attachment & Loss: VII: Separation and Anger*. New York: Basic Books.

Bradbury, R. (1950). *The Martian Chronicles*. New York: William Morrow.

Bradbury, R. (1953). *Fahrenheit 451*. New York: Simon & Schuster.

Brothers Grimm. (1972). *The Complete Grimm's' Fairy Tales*. M. Hunt & J. Stern (Trans.). New York: Pantheon Books.

Brucks, D., & von Bayern, A. (2020). Parrots voluntarily help each other to obtain food rewards. *Current Biology*, 30: 292–297.

Bunyan, J. (1678). *The Pilgrim's Progress*. New York: Dover Publications, 2003.

Burns, K., Hutton, I., & Shepherd, L. (2021). Primitive eusociality in a land plant. *Ecology*. 10: 1002.

Camus, A. (1947). *The Plague*. Paris: Gallimard.

Capellini, I., Barton, R., McNamara, P., & Preston, B. (2010). *Evolution of Sleep: Phylogenetic and Functional Perspectives*. London: Cambridge University Press.

Choi, J., Cutler, A., & Broersma, M. (2017). Early development of abstract language knowledge: Evidence from perception-production transfer of birth-language memory. *Royal Society Open Science*, 4: 160–166.

Chomsky, N. (1959). Review of B. F. Skinner's verbal behavior. *Language*, 35: 26–58.

Chomsky, N. (1965). *Aspects of the Theory of Syntax*. Cambridge, MA: MIT Press.

Chomsky, N. (1978). *Syntactic Structures*. Berlin: Mouton.

Collins, D. (1976). *The Human Evolution: From Ape to Artist*. New York & London: Penguin/Random house.

Cosans, C. (2009). *Owen's Ape & Darwin's Bulldog: Beyond Darwinism and Creationism*. Bloomington: Indiana University Press.

Crichton, M. (1969). *The Andromeda Strain*. New York: Knopf.

Crick, F. (1994). *The Astonishing Hypothesis: The Scientific Search for the Soul*. New York: Charles Scribner's Sons.

Darwin, C. (1859). *On the Origin of Species*. London: John Murray.

Darwin, C. (1871). *The Descent of Man, and Selection in Relation to Sex*. London: Forgotten Books (2015).

Dawkins, R. (1976). *The Selfish Gene*. Oxford: Oxford University Press.

de Waal, F. (2016). *Are We Smart Enough to Know How Smart Animals Are?* New York: W. W. Norton.

de Waal, F. (2019). *Mama's Last Hug. Animal Emotions and What They Tell Us about Ourselves*. New York WW. Norton Company.

Descartes, R. (1637). *Discourse on Method and Meditations on First Philosophy*. Cress, D. (Trans.). 4th Ed., 1999.

Diamond, J. (1997). *Guns, Germs and Steel*. New York: Norton.

Dobzhansky, T. (1937). *Genetics and the Origin of Species*. Columbia University Biological Series, V. 11. New York: Columbia University Press.

Dollard, J., Miller, N., Dood, L., Mowrer, O., & Sears, R. (1944). *Frustration and Aggression*. London: Kegan, Paul, Trench, Trubner & Co.

Durkheim, E. (1895). *Rules of Sociological Method*. New York: Free Press (1982).

Durkin, K., Rutter, D., & Tucker, H. (1982). Social interaction and language acquisition: Motherese help you. *First Language*, 3: 107–120.

Edgerton, R. (1992). *Sick Societies*. New York: Free Press.

Eliade, M. (1964). *Shamanism: Archaic Techniques of Ecstasy.* New York: Pantheon Books.
Everett, D. (2005). Cultural constraints on grammar and cognition in Piraha: Another look at the design features of human language. *Current Anthropology*, 46: 621–646.
Everett, D. (2008). *Don't Sleep, There Are Snakes: Life and Language in the Amazon Jungle.* New York: Pantheon Books.
Fagles, R. (trans.) (1990). *Iliad.* New York: Viking-Penguin.
Fagles, R. (trans.) (1996). *Odyssey.* New York: Viking-Penguin.
Ferguson, C. (1964). Baby talk in six languages. *American Anthropologist,* 66: 103–114.
Fernald, A. (1996). The onset of language development. In: P. Bloom (Ed.). *Language Acquisition: Core Readings.* Cambridge, MA: MIT Press. pp. 51–94.
Fernald, A., & Kuhl, P. (1987). Acoustic determinants of infant preference for motherese speech. *Infant Behavior & Development,* 10: 279–293.
Frances, A. (2014). *Saving Normal: An Insider's Revolt against Out-of-Control Psychiatric Diagnosis, DSM-5, Big Pharma, and the Medicalization of Ordinary Life.* New York: William Morrow.
Freud, S. (1900). *The Interpretation of Dreams. S.E.,* 4–5. London: Hogarth Press.
Freud, S. (1911). *Formulations on the Two Principles of Mental Functioning. S.E.,* 12. London: Hogarth Press.
Freud, S. (1914). *Thoughts in Times of War and Death. S.E.,* 14: 273–300. London: Hogarth Press.
Freud, S. (1915). *The Unconscious. S.E.,* 14: 166–215. London: Hogarth Press.
Freud, S. (1920). *Beyond the Pleasure Principle. S.E.,* 18: 3–68. London: Hogarth Press.
Freud, S. (1930). *Civilization and Its Discontents. S.E.,* 21: 59–148. London: Hogarth Press.
Freud, S., & Bullitt, W. (1967). *Thomas Woodrow Wilson: A Psychological Study.* New York: Houghton-Mifflin.
Freud, S., & Einstein, A. (1933). *Why War? S.E.,* 22: 197–210. London: Hogarth Press.
Fromm, E. (1973). *The Anatomy of Human Destructiveness.* New York: Holt, Rinehart & Winston.
Fromm-Reichmann, F. (1948). Notes on the development of treatment of schizophrenics by psychoanalytic psychotherapy. *Psychiatry,* 11: 265–273.
Fromm-Reichmann, F. (1952). Some aspects of psychoanalytic psychotherapy with schizophrenics. In E. Brody & F. Redlich (Eds.) *Psychotherapy with Schizophrenics* (pp. 89–111). New York: International Universities Press.
Frost, R. (1967). Stopping by woods (224), and the road not taken (105). In E. Lathem (Ed.) *The Poetry of Robert Frost.* New York: Holt, Rhinehart & Winston.
Gallup, G. (1970). Chimpanzees: Self-recognition. *Science,* 67: 86–87.
Gallup, G. (1977). Self-recognition in primates: A comparative approach to the bidirectional properties of consciousness. *American Psychologist,* 329,338.
Gallup, G. (1982). Self-awareness and the emergence of mind in primates. *Journal of Primatology,* 2: 237–248.
Gardner, R. A., & Gardner, B. (1998). *The Structure of Learning from Sign Stimuli to Sign Language.* Hillsdale, NJ: Lawrence Erlbaum Associates.
Gardner, R. A., Gardner, B., & Van Cantfort, T. (1989). *Teaching Sign Language to Chimpanzees.* New York: SUNY Press.
Gibson, R. (1989). The application of psychoanalytic principles to the hospitalized patient. In A. Silver (Ed.) *Psychoanalysis and Psychosis* (pp. 183–206). Madison, CT: International Universities Press.

Gintis, H. (2011). Gene-culture evolution and the nature of human sociality. *Philosophical Transactions B of the Royal London Biological Society*, 366: 878–888.
Goodall, J. (1986). *The Chimpanzees of Gombe: Patterns of Behavior.* New York: Belknap Press.
Goodall, J., & Berman, P. (1999). *Reason for Hope: A Spiritual Journey.* New York: Grand Central Publishing.
Goodall, J., & Wrangham, R. (2010). *In the Shadow of Man.* Boston. MA: Mariner Books.
Gould, S. J. (1977). *Ontogeny and Phylogeny.* Cambridge, MA: Harvard University Press.
Graeber, D., & Wengrow, D. (2021). *The Dawn of Everything: A New Theory of Humanity.* New York: Farrar, Straus & Giroux.
Greenspan, S., & Shanker, S. (2005). *The First Idea: How Symbols, Language and Intelligence Evolved from Our Primate Ancestors to Modern Humans.* Cambridge, MA: Da Capo Press.
Grieser, D., & Kuhl, P. (1988). Maternal speech to infants in a tonal language: Support for universal prosodic features in motherese. *Developmental Psychology*, 24: 14–20.
Haberman, M. (2022) *Confidence Man: The Making of Donald Trump and the Breaking of America.* New York, NY: Penguin.
Harari, Y. N. (2011). *Sapiens: A Brief History of Humankind.* New York: Harper.
Hayes, C., & Hull, D. (Eds.) (2001), *Selection Theory and Social Construction: The Evolutionary Naturalistic Epistemology of Donald T. Campbell.* (SUNY series in Philosophy and Biology). New York: Suny Press.
Heijmans, B., Tobi, E., Stein, A., et al. (2008). Persistent epigenetic differences associated with prenatal exposure to famine in humans. *Proceeds of the National Academy of Science*, 105: 17046–17049.
Henrich, J. (2015). *The Secret of Our Success: How Culture Is Driving Human Evolution, Domesticating Our Species, and Making Us Smarter.* Princeton, NJ: Princeton University Press.
Hoffman, L. (2003). Mother's ambivalence with their babies and toddlers: Manifestations of conflicts with aggression. *Journal of the American Psychoanalytic Association*, 51: 1219–1240.
Huxley, A. (1932). *Brave New World.* London: Chatto & Windus. New York: Harper (2017).
Hyman, S. (2013). Post on website of Dana Foundation.
Ilitis, H. (1924). *Life of Mendel.* E. & C. Paul (Trans.). New York: Norton (1932).
Insel, T. (2013). Post on website of National Institute of Mental Health.
Insel, T. (2022). *Healing: O:ur Path from Mental Illness to Mental Health.* London: Penguin Press.
Jaynes, J. (1976). *The Origin of Consciousness in the Breakdown of the Bicameral Mind.* New York: Houghton Mifflin.
Johnson, J., & Newport, E. (1989). Critical period effects in second language learning: the influence of maturation state on the acquisition of English as a second language. *Cognitive Psychology*, 21:60–99.
Joseph, J. (2003). *The Gene Illusion: Genetic Research in Psychiatry and Psychology under the Microscope.* Herefordshire: PCCS Books.
Jung, C. G. (1912). Two kinds of thinking. In *Symbols of Transformation.* Bollingen Series XX V. 5, F. R. C. Hull (Trans.). New York. *The Basic Writings of C. G. Jung.* V. De Laszlo (Ed.). New York: The Modern Library (1959), pp. 10–36.

Jung, C. G. (1968). *Man and His Symbols.* New York: Dell.

Jung, C. G. (1981). The archetypes and the collective unconscious. The archetypes and the collective unconscious. In: *Collected Works of C.G. Jung.* V, 9, Part I. Princeton, NJ: Princeton University Press.

Kahneman, D. (2011). Thinking *Fast and Slow.* New York: Farrar, Straus & Giroux.

Kant, I. (1787, 1798). *The Critique of Pure Reason.*

King, S. (1978). *The Stand.* New York: Doubleday.

Klein, M. (1928). Early stages of the Oedipus Complex. *International Journal of Psychoanalysis,* 9: 167–180.

Klein, M. (1946). Notes on some schizoid mechanisms. In: Klein, M., Envy and Gratitude and other works, 1946–1963. London: Hogarth Press, pp. 1–24.

Knox, B. (1990). Introduction. In R. Fagles (Trans.) *Iliad.* New York: Viking-Penguin, pp. 1–72.

Kolata, G. (1984). Studying learning in the womb. *Science,* 225: 302–303.

Kolbert, E. (2014). *The Sixth Extinction.* New York: Henry Holt.

Kolbert, E. (2021). *Under a White Sky.* New York: Crown.

Lamarck, J. (1809). *Philosophie Zoologique.* Philosophie zoologique ou exposition des considérations relatives à l'histoire naturelle des animaux. Paris: Musee de Histoire Naturelle.

Lancet Commission on Pollution and Health, October, 2017. Open access. https://www.thelancet.com/commissions/pollution-and-health

Lévy-Bruhl, L. (1923). *Primitive Mentality.* New York: AMS Press (1978).

Lévy-Bruhl, L. (1928). *The Soul of the Primitive.* New York: Routledge (2016).

Lévy-Bruhl, L. (1935). *Primitive Mythology.* Brisbane: University of Queensland Press, 1983.

Lifton, R. (2017). *The Nazi Doctors: Medical Killing and the Psychology of Genocide.* New York: Basic Books.

Lifton, R. J. (1961). *Thought Reform and the Psychology of Totalism: A Study of "Brainwashing" in China.* New York: Norton.

Linnaeus, C. (1735). *Systema Naturae.* Netherlands.

Lorenz, K. (1966). *On Aggression.* New York: Routledge (1996).

Lyons-Ruth, K. (2003). Dissociation and the parent-infant dialogue. *Journal of the American Psychoanalytic Association,* 51: 883–911.

Mahler, M. (1968). *On Human Symbiosis and the Vicissitudes of Individuation: V.I: Infantile Psychosis.* New York: International Universities Press.

Mahler, M., Bergman, A., & Pine, F. (1975). *The Psychological Birth of the Human Infant: Symbiosis and Individuation.* New York: Basic Books.

Main, M. (1977). The ultimate causation of some infant attachment phenomena. *Behavioral and Brain Science,* 2: 640–643.

Main, M. (2000). The organized categories of infant, child, and adult attachment: Flexible vs. inflexible attention under attachment-related stress. *Journal of the American Psychoanalytic Association,* 48: 1055–1096.

Malgrange, B., & Nguyen, R. (2022). Scaling brain neurogenesis across evolution. *Science.* Epub, 1155–1156.

Mandelbrot, B. (1967). How long is the coast of Britain? Statistical self-similarity and fractional dimension. *Science,* 155: 636–638.

Martin, B. (1982). Critique of nuclear extinction. *Journal of Peace Research,* 19: 287–300.

Masataka, N. (1996). Perception of motherese in a signed language by 6-month-old *deaf* infants. *Developmental Psychology,* 32(5), 874–879.

May, R., Lawton, J., & Stork, N. (1995). Assessing extinction rates. In J. Lawton & R. May (Eds.) *Extinction Rates* (pp. 1–24). Oxford: Oxford University Press.

Mayr, E. (1963). *Animal Species and Evolution*. Cambridge, MA: Belknap Press of Harvard University Press.

Mayr, E. (1970). *Populations, Species and Evolution*. Cambridge: Belknap Press of Harvard University Press.

Melville, H. (1851). *Moby Dick*. New York: Harper & Brothers.

Mendel, G. (1866). *Experiments on Plant Hybridization*. Lulu.com (2018).

Mesoudi, A., & Thornton, A. (2018). What is cumulative cultural evolution? *Proceedings of Biological Science*, Open Access Journal 13 June.

Morel, B. (1860). *Etudes Cliniques, V.II: Traité des maladies mentales*. Paris: J.B. Bailliere.

Nibert, D. (2013). *Animal Oppression and Human Violence: Domesecration, Capitalism, and Global Conflict*. New York: Columbia University Press.

Nicholson, S. (Ed.) (1987). *Shamanism*. Wheaton, IL: The Theosophical Publishing House.

Novacek, M., & Wheeler, Q. (1992). *Extinction and Phylogeny*. New York: Columbia.

Ord, T. (2020). *The Precipice: Existential Risk and the Future of Humanity*. New York: Hachette Books.

Owen, R. (1860). Darwin on the Origin of Species. *Edinburgh Review*3: 487–532.

Panksepp, J., & Biven, L. (2012). *The Archeology of Mind: Neuroevolutionary Origins of Human Emotions*. New York: W.W. Norton.

Partanan, E., Kujala, F., Naatanin, R., Lutola, A., Sambeth, A., & Huotilainen, N. (2013). Learning induced neuroplasticity in speech before birth. *Proceedings of the American Academy of Sciences*, 110: 15145–15150.

Partanen, E., & Virtala, P. (2017). Prenatal sensory development. In B. Hopkins, E. Geangu, & S. Linkenauger (Eds.) *The Cambridge Encyclopedia of Child Development* (pp. 231–241). Cambridge: Cambridge University Press.

Patterson, F. (1980). In search of man: Experiments in primate communication. *Michigan Quarterly Review*, 19: 1–15.

Paul, R. (2015). *Mixed Messages; Cultural and Genetic Inheritance in the Constitution of Human Society*. Chicago, IL: University of Chicago Press.

Paus, T., Zijdembos, A., Worsele, K., Collins, L., Blumenthal, J., Geidd, J., Rapoport, J., Evans A., et al. (1999). Structural maturation of neural pathways in children and adolescents: In vivo study. *Science*, 283: 1908–1911.

Piaget, J. (1936). *The Origins of Intelligence in Children*. New York: International Universities Press (1952).

Pimentel, D., and M. Giampietro (1994). Implications of the Limited Potential of Technology to Increase the Carrying Capacity of Our Planet. *Human Ecology Review* Summer/Autumn, 1: 248–251.

Pinker, S. (1994). *The Language Instinct: How the Mind Creates Language*. New York: William Morrow & Co.

Pinker, S. (2018). *Enlightenment Now: The Case for Reason, Science, Humanism and Progress*. New York: Viking.

Pinson A., Xing L., Namba T., Kalebic N., Peters J., Oegema C.E., Traikov S., Reppe K., Riesenberg S., Maricic T., et al. (2022). Human TKTL1 implies greater neurogenesis in frontal neocortex of modern humans than Neanderthals. *Science*, 377: 1105–1107.

Richerson, P., & Boyd, R. (2006). *Not by Genes Alone: How Culture Transformed Human Evolution*. Chicago, IL: University of Chicago Press.

Rivera-Gaxiola, M., Silvia-Pereyra, J., & Kuhl, P. (2005). Brain potentials to native and non-native speech: Contrasts in 7- and 11-month-old American infants. *Developmental Science*, 8:162–172.

Robbins, M. (2011). *The Primordial Mind in Health and Illness: A Cross-Cultural Perspective*. London & New York: Routledge.

Robbins, M. (2015). The "royal road" – to what? *The Annual of Psychoanalysis*, 38: 196–214.

Robbins, M. (2018a). The primary process: Freud's profound yet neglected contribution to the psychology of consciousness. *Psychoanalytic Inquiry*, 38: 186–197.

Robbins, M. (2018b). *Consciousness, Language and Self: Psychoanalytic, Linguistic and Anthropological Explorations of the Dual Nature of Mind*. London & New York: Routledge.

Robbins, M. (2019). *Psychoanalysis Meets Psychosis: Attachment, Separation, and the Undifferentiated Unintegrated Mind*. London & New York: Routledge.

Robbins, M. (in press). *What Makes Humans Unique: Evolution and the Two Structures of the Mind*. London & New York: Routledge.

Robertson, J., & Robertson, J. (1971). Young children in brief separation – A fresh look. *Psychoanalytic Study of the Child*, 26: 264–315.

Savage-Rumbaugh, S. (2001). *Apes, Language and the Human Mind*. London: Oxford University Press.

Schwab, K., Groh, T., Schwab, M., & Witte, H. (2009). Nonlinear analysis and modeling of cortical activation and deactivation patterns in the immature fetal electrocorticogram. *Chaos: An Interdisciplinary Journal of Nonlinear Science*, 19(1): 015111.

Segal, H. (1993). On the clinical usefulness of the concept of death instinct. *The International Journal of Psychoanalysis*, 74: 55–61.

Selye, H. (1946). *The Stress of Life*. New York: McGraw-Hill.

Shakespeare, W. (2005). Julius Caesar Act I, Scene III, 140-141. In S. Wells, et al. (Eds.) *The Oxford Shakespeare*. London: Oxford University Press.

Sharpless, E. (1985). Identity formation as reflected in the acquisition of personal pronouns. *Journal of the American Psychoanalytic Association*, 71: 861–885.

Shelley, M. (1818). *Frankenstein, or the Modern Prometheus*. Independently published (2017).

Shute, N. (1957). *On the Beach*. London: Heinemann.

Shweder, R. (2009). Has Piaget been upstaged? A reply to Hallpike. *American Anthropologist*, 87: 138–144.

Simon, B. (1978). *Mind and Madness in Ancient Greece: The Classical Roots of Modern Psychiatry*. Ithaca, NY: Cornell University Press.

Snell, B. (1982). *The Discovery of the Mind: The Greek Origins of European Thought*. New York: Andesite Press.

Solomon, S., Greenberg, J., & Pyszczynski, T. (2015). *The Worm at the Core: On the Role of Death in Life*. New York: Random House.

Sophocles (2000). *The Three Theban Plays*. R. Fagles (trans.). New York: Penguin Classics (2000).

Terrace, H. (1979). *Nim*. New York: Knopf.

Terrace, H. (2019). *Why Chimpanzees Can't Learn Language and Only Humans Can*. New York: Columbia University Press.
Topol, E. (2019). Op-Ed March 11 *New York Times*.
Trevarthen, C. (2005). First things first: Infants make good use of the sympathetic rhythm of imitation, without reason or language. *Journal of Child Psychotherapy*, 31: 91–113.
Trisos, C., Merow, C., & Pigot, A. (2020). The projected timing of abrupt disruption from climate change. *Nature*. Published on line 8 April.
Trump, M. (2020). *Too Much and Not Enough*. New York: Simon & Schuster.
van den Dungen, W. (2019). *Ancient Egyptian Writings*. Lulu.com (self-published).
Vico, G. (1744). *Principi Scienza Nuova*. Naples: Stamperia Muziana.
Virsida, A. R. (2001). The Death Drive: Psychic Construction or Destruction? *Psychoanalytic Review*, 88: 511–523.
Von Bertalanffy, L. (1952). *Problems of Life*. New York: John Wiley & Sons.
Vonnegut, K. (1963). *Cat's Cradle*. New York: Holt, Rhinehart & Winston.
Weiss, E. (1942). Psychic defence and the technique of its analysis. *International Journal of Psycho-Analysis*, 23: 69–80.
Werker, J., & Tees, R. (1984). Cross-language speech perception: Evidence for perceptual reorganization during the first year of life. *Infant Behavior and Development*, 7: 49–63.
Wilson, E. O. (1975). *Sociobiology: A New Synthesis*. Cambridge, MA: Harvard University Press/Belknap Press.
Wilson, E. O. (2012). *The Social Conquest of Earth*. London: Liveright Publishing.
Winnicott, D. W. (1949). Hate in the countertransference. *International Journal of Psycho-Analysis*, 30: 69–74.
Winnicott, D. W. (1951). Transitional objects and transitional phenomena. In *Collected Papers* (pp. 229–242). London: Tavistock (1958).
Winnicott, D. W. (1960). Ego distortion in terms of true and false self. In D. W. Winnicott (Ed.) (1965). *The Maturational Processes and the Facilitating Environment*. London: Hogarth, pp. 140–152.

INDEX

For Product Safety Concerns and Information please contact our EU representative GPSR@taylorandfrancis.com
Taylor & Francis Verlag GmbH, Kaufingerstraße 24, 80331 München, Germany

www.ingramcontent.com/pod-product-compliance
Ingram Content Group UK Ltd.
Pitfield, Milton Keynes, MK11 3LW, UK
UKHW020138200926
475702UK00005B/813